THE

BIG BOOK OF

HORMONES

THE BIG BOOK OF HORMONES

SILOAM

Most CHARISMA HOUSE BOOK GROUP products are available at special quantity discounts for bulk purchase for sales promotions, premiums, fund-raising, and educational needs. For details, write Charisma House Book Group, 600 Rinehart Road, Lake Mary, Florida 32746, or telephone (407) 333-0600.

THE BIG BOOK OF HORMONES by Siloam
Published by Siloam
Charisma Media/Charisma House Book Group
600 Rinehart Road
Lake Mary, Florida 32746
www.charismahouse.com

Cover design by Lisa Rae McClure
Design Director: Justin Evans

For more information on books published by Siloam, visit www.charismahouse.com.

This book contains the opinions and ideas of its authors. It is solely for informational and educational purposes and should not be regarded as a substitute for professional medical treatment. The nature of your body's health condition is complex and unique. Therefore, you should consult a health professional before you begin any new exercise, nutrition, or supplementation program or if you have questions about your health. Neither the authors nor the publisher shall be liable or responsible for any loss or damage allegedly arising from any information or suggestion in this book.

Library of Congress Cataloging-in-Publication Data:

The big book of hormones : survival secrets to naturally eliminate hot flashes, regulate your moods, improve your memory, lose weight, sleep better, and more! / [edited by] Siloam.

    pages cm

  Summary: "End the hormone roller coaster ride for good. Women want to look younger and live longer, have more vibrant and balanced lives all while making "it" happen like superwoman. Using the wealth of resources from Siloam's most popular health writers, including Janet Maccaro, Don Colbert, Reginald Cherry, Cherie Calbom, and Scott Farhart, The Big Book of Hormones gives readers a comprehensive book on women's hormone health that covers topics such as anti-aging, weight loss, natural health (supplements, vitamins, superfoods, smoothies, and juices), stress management, and more. Women will learn: How to identify hormone imbalances When to go to the doctor The best protocols for restoration, weight loss, sleep, memory recall, regulating mood swings, and preventing other diseases related to hormone depletion such as heart disease, osteoporosis, certain cancers, and more"-- Provided by publisher.

  ISBN 978-1-62998-207-6 (paperback) -- ISBN 978-1-62998-584-8 (e-book)

  1. Hormone therapy. 2. Women--Health and hygiene. I. Siloam (Publisher)

  RM286.B54 2015

  615.3'6--dc23

2015003009

15 16 17 18 19 — 987654321
Printed in the United States of America

CONTENTS

we are beautifully and wonderfully made.

Introduction

BEAUTIFULLY AND WONDERFULLY MADE

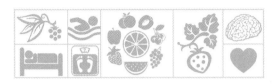

I will praise You, for you made me with fear and wonder;
marvelous are Your works, and You know me completely.
—PSALM 139:14

O N SOMEONE'S BIRTHDAY we may quote a passage such as this one. But do we believe it, really, in our own lives—especially as we face the inevitable passage of the years? Do you believe that the way you look and feel today is as beautiful or as wonderful as in the past? You may look back even a decade and wonder what became of that vibrant, smiling young woman you used to be. You have weathered many storms, and now you can trace their history in your body. Those adult responsibilities, choices, habits, and traumas have taken a definite toll.

Behind the scenes your hormones have played a huge role where your health and well-being are concerned. So much depends on them, just as their functioning depends on many other aspects of your life. Everything is interdependent. Despite a woman's tendency to ruefully bemoan her hormones, especially at a certain time of the month, she knows that God invented hormones and He knew what He was doing. He designed their intricate dances within your body. He also designed your mind to be able to understand how to live in and maintain a body that may, at times, seem to belong to someone else.

Victim or Survivor?

As a population of women gets older, two distinct groups emerge: victims and survivors. Both groups may have experienced roughly the same amount of sorrow and pain in their lives, but their views on their experiences prove to be dramatically different. Victims become stuck, paralyzed by the past, unable to forgive and move forward. Survivors, on the other hand, have learned from the past and use it to propel them forward using the wisdom they've gained and the spiritual growth they've experienced as inspiration to continue on, with faith and hope as their traveling companions.

The older you get, the more important this mature wisdom becomes. "Aging" does not have to be an unwelcome word. You can learn as you go to manage every aspect of your hormonally driven life: your dietary and health concerns, spiritual and emotional growth, maturity issues, and more. In fact, you can define the aging process to include personalized refinements that benefit your own unique body, mind, and spirit.

A woman's life is filled with the joy of many wonderful seasons, according to a wise Creator's design. The Word of God says, "To everything there is a season, a time for every purpose under heaven" (Eccles. 3:1). In the springtime a woman's femininity awakens in the tender bloom of her youth. In the summer her fruitful body fills her life with the busy joy of babies and children. But the autumn of a woman's life can be the most wonderful season of all. During the years of menopause, a harvest of all the good things a woman has planted into those around her comes back to her. In addition, the joy of grown-up children, grandchildren, and the freedom of new pursuits can paint her life with a burst of change as beautiful and as varied as a dazzling display of autumn color.

God's desire for you as you pass through the natural life transitions of postpuberty, premenopause, menopause, and postmenopause is to be healthy and renewed, as the psalmist declares, "He fills my life with good things. My youth is renewed like the eagle's!" (Ps. 103:5, NLT).

Steward of a Precious Gift

You can add up the statistics on average life spans and speculate about factors in the biological aging process, but what does that tell you about *your* life? Each of us has been given a predetermined number of days on this earth, and each one of these days is a gift. How are you treating this precious gift? Are you disrespecting it by not caring for your body or nurturing your soul? Or are you living intentionally, realizing that you have a responsibility to be the very best expression of life that you can be?

At the end of our days all of us want to have run the good race and to have fought the good fight. We want to have made a difference while on our earthly journey. We want to leave a "footprint" (a "heartprint," so to speak) as proof that we were alive and that we mattered to those we loved.

This is where stewardship comes in. What will you do with your appointed days? Will you embrace each one, the good and bad, the dark with the bright? Each day, whatever the circumstances of it, has been given to teach you, grow you, mature and refine you, bring you joy, and give you the ability to be compassionate, loving, and forgiving. In other words, you are being fired in the kiln of life. How will you come forth at the end? Will you come to the end of your days with a life as beautiful as the finest porcelain? Or will you instead arrive cracked and broken, lacking a testimony or legacy of happiness?

If you look back on your life and see that you haven't lived it the best, you can begin right now to experience a richer life filled with better health, more stable emotions, and a deeper spiritual walk. You can expect not only to live a long life, but also to live better at any stage and any age. You can learn ways to bring health to your earthly frame, ways to heal your emotions, and ways to bring you closer to your Creator.

There is a balance in nature that is so delicately and intricately interdependent that it is beyond the scope of our understanding. Yet when that balance is lost, we can immediately see the outcome. As rainfall decreases, aquatic plants die due to lowered water levels, fish die because of poor oxygenation, animals on the water's edge leave or die from starvation, and insect populations increase as birds and other natural feeders leave the ecosystem, leaving it desolate and compromised. The same holds true for a woman's body. Once balance is lost, her quality of life is never the same. She ceases to flourish, and her dreams of vibrant and abundant health are replaced with fatigue, loss of mental clarity, anxiety, depression, and degenerative disease.

But a woman who has learned—usually from personal experience and often the hard way—how to balance her service to others with her care for herself, her hard work with her relaxation and play, her emotional needs with her mental and physical needs, and even how to balance her healthy weight on the bathroom scale, has learned more than most women ever do.

A woman who has achieved balance is free from anxiety, depression, worry, and physical maladies. Sleep refreshes her, vibrancy abounds, and the lives of the people around her are enriched by her wisdom and ability to weather life's storms with grace and dignity.

A balanced woman is a treasure to behold. Her beauty transcends the physical realm. Her strength and insight shine forth as a beacon to others. Her body, mind, and spirit function in concert. She walks in abundant and divine health. A balanced woman gives and nurtures unconditionally, but at the same time she knows the love she gives so freely needs to be given to herself as well. She knows that she is worthy of love and care. A woman's body, when in balance, allows her to be the full expression of what God designed her to be! Finding your balance is worth the effort.

Year After Year

It is truly possible to keep moving through the decades of your life, even when significant new challenges arise, with joyfulness and vibrancy. A Christian woman has gained an edge on the people who have not embraced Jesus Christ as Lord and Savior. After all, He is the one who said, "I am the way, the truth, and the life" (John 14:6).

A newborn baby girl in the United States can expect to live well over eighty years. Whether those years are filled with anxious struggle and increased debilitation or one joyful victory after another depends entirely on a woman's connection to the source of life.

The matter at hand, regarding the topic of this book, is living life to the fullest as far as your hormones are concerned. Take a look at the table of contents. The chapter titles tell you at a glance what each chapter is about. Every chapter features an array of sidebars, charts, lists, and self-tests to enable you to get to know yourself better and also to anticipate and field the hormonal curve balls that may be coming your way in the years ahead. You can skip to the chapters that speak best to your current needs, and you can refer back to the book as your hormonal needs change.

 You may surprise yourself, especially if you have grown accustomed to suffering from hormonal imbalances. With a little help from your friends, you can learn not only how to survive, but also to *thrive!* Your life this year can be a new beginning for your eternal adventure of joy.

Chapter 1

WE'RE ALL WOMEN HERE

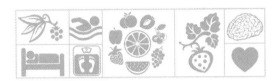

A S A WOMAN, you are a designer edition. When God designed you, He created someone very unique, just as special as the first woman He ever made. You know the story: "Then the rib which the LORD God had taken from man, He made into a woman, and He brought her to the man. Then Adam said, 'This is now bone of my bones and flesh of my flesh; she shall be called Woman, for she was taken out of Man'" (Gen. 2:22–23).

Interestingly, although the Bible states that females are formed from males, a developing fetus will automatically take a female form if not influenced early on by the male hormone testosterone. It is testosterone that closes the vagina, makes the labia turn into a scrotum, and elongates the clitoris to form a penis. Without it, a normal-appearing female will be formed, complete with breast development and a vagina, even if that person has the chromosomes of a male. So being female is no "accident" or "mistake."

Hormones for Life

The ovaries are the dominant organs in women. Nearly all of the sex hormones come from the ovaries, and they hold the key to much of what it means to be female. These almond-size oval structures are located on each side of the uterus. They produce the female sex hormones estrogen and progesterone, and they store all of the eggs needed for later reproduction. Each month dozens of eggs compete with each other to select the one egg that will be released for fertilization in a process called ovulation. In a complex interaction between the brain and the ovaries, one dominant egg reaches maturity and is released into the pelvic cavity where the fallopian tube takes it into itself. There one of the waiting sperm fertilizes it. The resulting new embryo journeys into the uterus to begin its new life.

The ovaries make a hormone called estrogen. From the onset of puberty to menopause, the ovaries produce this hormone daily. It's what keeps the female voice high, develops breasts, grows a uterine lining for later use in reproduction, and changes the shape of the pelvic bones to accommodate pregnancy. This hormone has been found to interact with almost every organ of the body in a powerful way. It causes calcium to bind to bone (the loss of estrogen is the primary cause of osteoporosis in women). It increases the good cholesterol and lowers the bad cholesterol, delaying the onset of heart attack and stroke in women compared to men. And this doesn't include the effects of estrogen on the brain.

When the egg is released in the middle of the menstrual cycle, a second hormone, called progesterone, is made. Its principle job is to prepare the uterine lining to receive an embryo. Without this preparation, the embryo would float by and fall out of the cervix, never implanting and never causing pregnancy. If an embryo does not implant and signal its existence to the ovary, the progesterone levels will fall and the uterine lining will tear away, beginning the familiar process of menstruation.

Puberty marks the physical, emotional, and sexual transition from childhood to adulthood. This transition occurs gradually and contains a series of well-defined events and milestones. The brain contains two structures—the hypothalamus and pituitary gland—that are responsible for turning on and regulating the secretion of hormones from the ovaries in women (the gonads). This is referred to as the hypothalamic-pituitary-gonadal axis and is initially active in the fetus and during the first few years following birth. It then becomes inactive until the onset of pubertal development. At approximately age eight the adrenal glands send a signal that turns on the gonadal sex hormone production approximately two years later. The process of pubertal development requires approximately four years to achieve full sexual maturation.

You do not want to live without hormones. Considering that hormones were not even discovered until the early 1900s, it should be no surprise that we are only now uncovering information about their good and bad effects. Basically hormones are signaling messengers involved in almost every chemical process in our bodies. They influence growth, metabolism, strength, endurance, and vitality. Hormones even control other hormones. Keeping them in a balance appropriate for one's age and stage in life increases your chance of good health and well-being.

Hormones Define a Woman's Seasons of Life

Any time after puberty a healthy woman's body is able to conceive a child. Her hormones keep her monthly cycle going, but they remain behind the scenes. She may not think about her hormones much at all—unless they subject her to uncomfortable monthly symptoms of premenstrual syndrome. Whether or not she experiences PMS or bears a child, months and years go by, and a variety of other hormonal "issues" may occur. She may develop cancer or another major health problem.

All along, where there's life, there are hormones, not only the ones that get top billing in the information stream (estrogen in particular), but also all of the others that regulate metabolism, energy, and other life processes. (You can learn more about them in the next chapter, which discusses the endocrine system and its robust but delicate balance.)

Sometime in her fourth decade a woman may begin to notice a shift. Her monthly menstrual periods may become irregular, and every part of her body may seem to be letting go of youth. Eventually the monthly period is a thing of the past, and she can now define herself as "menopausal." The story is far from over, though, and her hormones, even though they may have staggered a bit (or a lot) through the years, keep doing what they were designed to do.

How a woman has lived her life will affect how she experiences menopause and her propensity for developing a disease. Most women are comfortable with the concept that procreation is not the sole reason for their existence. Ordinary and extraordinary women frequently experience renewed vitality and a redirected creative force after menopause.

Since menopause is not a disease, taking medicine to get over it should be unnecessary. Estrogen and progesterone define physical femininity and are instrumental for reproduction; they are no longer needed at high levels when that is no longer the body's agenda. The body wisely turns down reproductive hormonal function at a certain age, but continues producing the same hormones at levels below those that maintain fertility. There are many redundant systems—hormones are produced in the skin, brain, and fat from other precursor hormones when the ovaries are no longer the chief source.

A woman's perfect design was never to accommodate proliferative levels of hormones every day, every hour. Estrogen and progesterone wax and wane throughout the month, even releasing in a pulsing fashion throughout the day. This natural rhythm spares hormone-sensitive tissue such as the breast, uterus, vagina, and endometrium from continued exposure to these highly stimulating agents. Where is the wisdom in supplementing hormones outside the normal range of a woman's biological clock? How does the body cope? What systems are responsible for clearing unwanted hormones?

According to the US Census Bureau, more than fifty million women will be older than fifty-one by the year 2020. As many as five thousand of those women per day enter menopause. The average woman can expect to live a third of her life postmenopausal.

Estrogen and Friends

When estrogen is prescribed by a physician and taken as a pill, lozenge, or through the skin, it is called exogenous—from an outside source. You can also take in exogenous estrogen through the foods you eat and from chemicals to which you are exposed, such as pesticides that mimic hormones.

The estrogen you make in your body is known as endogenous. Before menstrual cycles stop completely, the depletion of egg follicles in the ovary results in a steady decline of estrogen, although its measurement in the bloodstream can vary considerably. (Estrogen is further identified as estradiol, which is active throughout a woman's reproductive years; estriol, predominant during pregnancy; estetrol, produced only during pregnancy; and estrone, the main circulating estrogen during menopause.)

After menopause the main source of estrogen is from conversion of a precursor hormone called androstenedione that is made in the adrenal gland. Obviously entering menopause with healthy adrenals is important. By the time a woman is well into her postmenopausal years, most estradiol is derived from testosterone, but the predominant estrogen in circulation remains estrone.

Breast tissue, the brain, bone, coronary arteries, and the lining of the uterus are prime sites for final conversion stages of estrogen. Whether this is good or bad depends on many things. A healthy wallop of estrogen converted in the bone is beneficial, while in other tissues, such as the breast, it can prove harmful. The level of estrogen production in various areas of the body increases with age and weight. Generally a person with more fat cells is going to produce more estrogen. Because a woman's need for estrogen continues, the divine architect of the body made sure estrogen production would carry on.

Once estrogen is produced, it must move around the body in order to enter target-tissue cells and induce biological activity. Only about 2 or 3 percent is free to roam about on its own. The majority of the free estrogen combines with "sex-hormone-binding globulin" (SHBG). SHBG is somewhat like a taxi, and if something alters the amount available, it will influence the quantity of free estrogen—just as pulling taxis out of service leaves people to get around on their own. This is important because when estrogen is riding in the taxi, it is unable to do its work.

Once estrogen has made its way around the body and prompted a cell to respond to the message it carries, it ultimately makes its way to the liver where it is broken down and bound to bile acids, excreted into the gastrointestinal tract, and finally eliminated as feces or through the kidneys as urine. If, however, a woman's bowel is inhabited by the wrong kind of bacteria, estrogen can be reabsorbed and passed through the liver again to begin another trek, with another opportunity to influence cellular metabolism. And if your intestinal tract is poorly functioning, estrogen may be reabsorbed at a level your body cannot manage, or it could allow an over-abundance back into your system.

When it comes to staying healthy or getting sick, research tells us that the way estrogen is broken down is more important than any gene you may be lucky or unlucky enough to have inherited. These breakdown products have significant biologic effects that in some cases may influence the safety and efficacy of the estrogen your body makes or that you add through what you eat or take medicinally.

Learning to Parallel Park

How estrogen affects a cell and sets into motion a series of good or bad events is determined by which form of estrogen it is, how the liver breaks it down, a woman's genes, cell chemistry, and the particular receptor to which it binds. A receptor is like a parking place. It is the literal spot on the cell where estrogen attaches. What happens when it parks is determined by proteins, pathways, and processes by which receptors interact. There are two types, alpha and beta, and several subtypes of each. This explains why the body can respond to the same hormone differently—the parking spots are different. For instance, when estradiol binds to the alpha receptor, it tells the cell to begin certain chemical reactions; when it binds to the beta receptor, the message activated is exactly the opposite of what it set in motion with the alpha receptor.[1] (Note: The alpha receptor was discovered in 1986, the beta in 1996. These dates remind us how very new estrogen science happens to be.)

The time estrogen spends in its preferred parking place determines the biologic activity and, with respect to hormone therapy, the potency of the prescribed hormone. Estrogen receptors will bind with other than free estrogen. Many toxins and plant cells can park at a receptor with varying affinity and action. This is why so much of the current pharmaceutical research on hormones is geared toward the development of selective estrogen receptor modulators—SERMs—designer drugs that can activate some but not all target cells.

In some cases when these designer drugs are used, estrogen action is blocked; in others it is stimulated. For example, the SERM raloxifene stimulates bone growth through its action at the estrogen receptor, but it does not have a proliferative effect on breast and endometrial tissue. However, in the brain it acts in an antiestrogen way, making it more difficult for blood vessels to constrict and dilate appropriately, which may cause a woman taking raloxifene to experience increased hot flashes.

Plant-derived isoflavones and lignans and their metabolites can be considered natural SERMs. Although often referred to as "phytoestrogens," their actions on the cell are not that of an estrogen. They function in an agonist/antagonist fashion, or as an "adaptogen." Adaptogens have a balancing effect on the body, working in whatever direction is needed, rather than having one fixed action.

N&4

> Accumulating evidence indicates it is not estrogen—as either estradiol or estrone—but estrogen metabolites that may be contributing to the health risks associated with estrogen during menstruation, at menopause, or with hormone replacement therapy.

Don't Forget About Progesterone

Like estrogen, a progestogen is mainly metabolized in the liver, secreted in the bile, and excreted in the feces. The endogenous version can be metabolized in the brain and activates a receptor that results in varying degrees of sedation. Because synthetic progestin is not converted in the same way, it is more likely to intensify mood disorders. Most hormone regimens commonly include synthetic progestins such as medroxy-progesterone acetate (MPA), a drug structurally related to progesterone, or norethindrone acetate, developed from the testosterone molecule. Progestins have been shown to increase breast density, and a few small studies have linked it with increasing breast cancer risk. In the uterus, however, it stops cell proliferation. There is great variation in absorption between patients. Natural (nature-identical or bioidentical) progesterone is sold over the counter in low doses that do not build bone or protect against hyperplasia (proliferation of cells). It is available in standardized doses by prescription from regular or compounding pharmacies.

The Role of Testosterone

Besides progestin, hormone therapies increasingly include testosterone with estrogen. Most of the testosterone a woman makes originates in the ovary and is only slightly reduced at menopause. Any drop that occurs just before or after menopause is primarily due to changes in adrenal secretion. If a woman has her ovaries removed, she may be unable to produce testosterone at suitable levels.

Two forms of exogenous testosterone are available—natural and synthetic. While most people automatically consider that "natural" makes anything better, in this case natural testosterone is poorly absorbed through the gastrointestinal tract in comparison to the synthetic version, methyltestosterone, which comes in a variety of forms including pills. Natural testosterone is available through injection or pellets, although patches are the latest development. Testosterone has specific receptors in target tissues—especially in the brain and bone. As with all the reproductive hormones, how they are utilized by an individual woman is highly variable.

Keeping the Balance, Year After Year

So what are you to do with this information? Understanding that estrogen, the primary female hormone, is essential to good female health, what does it mean to be hormonally dominant or deficient? When a woman's hormone levels are referred to as "estrogen dominant," it sounds as if she is so full of estrogen it should be leaking out her pores.

In truth, a woman can be estrogen dominant in her breast tissue, because of the many estrogen receptors located in the breast, while simultaneously being estrogen deficient and suffering from polycystic ovaries or severe bone loss. There are medical states and disease processes where these imbalances necessitate either the addition or exclusion of exogenous hormones. In most cases baseline laboratory values will support such a decision.

And taking hormones at the point in time when your body was designed to deactivate them can stress your body, requiring it to work hard to change estrogen into breakdown products—metabolites—that are safe. In healthy women the body persists in producing hormones at levels that are appropriate for a body that is winding down. Production continues, as we have mentioned, because the body has redundant systems. Their purpose is no longer to help you reproduce, but they are fully functioning and designed to keep you going for the next thirty or forty years.

In other words, hormone levels that are within the normal range of a menopausal woman—when you are a menopausal woman—do not dictate medicinal supplementation. Adding hormones for the purpose of restoring premenopausal levels is not what nature intended. Where is the wisdom in that? We are supposed to move beyond childbearing. Your body was designed to reproduce for three to four decades, not for a lifetime. For certain the plan was not to flood it with twenty-year-old hormone levels 100 percent of the time. To that end, it is not the single-handed work of declining hormones that alone defines the progress of aging. Your perfect design includes getting old.

Balance of Good News and Bad

The situation can seem somewhat overwhelming. How can you reconcile yourself both to the idea that your aging body is going to give you a hard time and that this is a welcome development? For one thing, you can learn about it. Armed with solid information—which must be accumulated over time—you can make sensible lifestyle decisions. You cannot change the basic design of your body nor too many of the circumstances in which you find yourself, but you can certainly maintain your body to the best of your ability and seek to achieve the satisfying inner harmony of maturity.

Someone who is maturing in chronological age should also be growing mentally, emotionally, and spiritually. The latter holds the master key to a life well lived. Your hormones will be best able to help your body and mind to flourish if your spirit is in touch with the master designer Himself, God.

He is not only your Creator but also your master physician. Therefore, you never need to feel that you are adrift in the world without hope for your future. Doctors are only human, and the medical community has limited options. Your ability to make wise choices is also imperfect. Often when your health is compromised in some way, your ability to think clearly is too. But God knows just what you need. It you turn to the One who created your body, He will help you. He created this world and all of the remedies available in it, and He sent His Son to bring wholeness to your body, mind, and spirit. He is powerful—and He is on your side. When you turn to Him, He will always be with you and give you the answer to your deepest needs.

The apostle Paul declared this wonderful reality: "For I am persuaded that neither death nor life, neither angels nor principalities nor powers, neither things present nor things to come, neither height nor depth, nor any other created thing, shall be able to separate us from the love of God, which is in Christ Jesus our Lord" (Rom. 8:38–39). Everyone will face a moment of crisis, a midnight hour, at some point in his or her life. For some, the moment comes sooner than for others, but rest assured, your moment will come. What will happen at that time? Will you know what to do? Will you know how to pray?

Often this happens during a serious health crisis. Then as with Jesus's disciples, you can say, "Lord, teach me to pray." (See Luke 11:1.) Jesus provided them with the pattern prayer that we still use today, the prayer called the Lord's Prayer. Jesus gave this prayer to His disciples—and to us today—not only for us to memorize and recite, but also to teach us the basic principles involved in praying. This simple prayer embodies certain fundamentals such as trust in God's guidance and provision and freedom from sin. Praying along those lines activates our relationship with our ever-loving, everlasting Father.

Five Ways to Pray for Your Physical Well-being

When you are concerned about a "female" matter, what is the first thing you should do? To whom should you turn? The psalmist declared, "God is our refuge and strength, a well-proven help in trouble" (Ps. 46:1). The psalms are filled with prayers from people who rejoiced when God heard their cries and delivered them. You may turn to their prayers and pray them in your hour of need as well, expecting your loving heavenly Father to answer you as well. But sometimes it is difficult to know exactly how to pray, especially when you are confused or worried. Here are four suggestions:

Pray for openness to hear God's voice.

You may be overwhelmed with unsolicited advice from well-meaning friends or loved ones. You may also face confusing decisions as to which tests or procedures to undergo or which medical options to pursue. Your doctor may be biased toward a certain treatment option and may be pressuring you to make decisions for which you feel unprepared. The first step to take at such a time is to pray for God's voice to cut through the din of all other voices and clearly make Himself and His will known.

Pray to know how to pray.

Sometimes the confusion can be so great that you may feel at a loss to know how to pray at all. The Holy Spirit is your heavenly guide—your instructor in the things of God (John 16:13). He is willing and available to show you how to pray. Begin to spend time waiting on God, and ask the Holy Spirit to give you the words to pray.

Pray for correct understanding of Scripture.

When you understand what God's Word has to say about your personal health, you will become more effective in your prayers. If you believe in salvation—through Christ's sacrifice on the cross to forgive your sins—then according to the Scriptures we must believe He cares about your physical well-being. The Bible declares of Christ's death: "He Himself took our infirmities and bore our sicknesses" (Matt. 8:17). The Bible also teaches us to persevere in prayer. (See Luke 18; Ephesians 6; Daniel 9.)

The Bible says, "Pray without ceasing" (1 Thess. 5:17). And again, "Pray in the spirit always with all kinds of prayer and supplication. To that end be alert with all perseverance and supplication" (Eph. 6:18). Be patient. Be faithful. Be determined. Keep praying and believing, and persevere until the answer comes.

Specifically target your prayers toward your personal situation.

Become informed about how your body works. Learn as many specifics as you can. Armed with as much information as you can gather, actively pray, using that information to your advantage. For instance, if your doctor tells you that a specific artery near your heart is becoming blocked and causing cardiovascular difficulties, then pray specifically for that particular artery, that it would become clear, in the name of Jesus! Or if there is a cancerous growth in your body, find out specifically where it is, and then continually lay your hands on that part of your body, commanding the cancer to shrink and disappear.

Pray for God to make clear His pathway that He has designed specifically for you. Bring the options that your doctor presents to you before the throne of grace, and ask the Father which way He would have you go. As you acknowledge Him, He will give you His peace and will guide you with His Holy Spirit into the way you should go.

Chapter 2

WHEN THINGS ARE OUT OF BALANCE

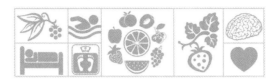

WHAT IS A hormone anyway? We may use names such as "estrogen," "testosterone," and "progesterone" as part of our everyday vocabulary, but do we really know what we're talking about?

Hormones are your body's chemical messengers.[1] They travel in your bloodstream to tissues or organs. They work slowly, over time, and affect many different processes, including:

NB&
- Growth and development
- Metabolism—how your body gets energy from the foods you eat
- Sexual function
- Reproduction
- Mood

Where Do Hormones Come From?

Endocrine glands, which are special groups of cells, make hormones. The major endocrine glands are the pituitary, pineal, thymus, thyroid, adrenal glands, and pancreas. In addition, men produce hormones in their testes, and women produce them in their ovaries.

The endocrine system is made up of the eight endocrine glands that not only produce and store hormones, but also secrete them. Although the major endocrine glands are scattered throughout the body, they are still considered to be one system because they have similar functions, similar mechanisms of influence, and many important interrelationships.[2]

Hormones are powerful. It takes only a tiny amount to cause big changes in cells or even your whole body. That is why having too much or too little of a certain hormone can be serious. Laboratory tests can measure the hormone levels in your blood, urine, or saliva.

Some glands also have non-endocrine regions that have functions other than hormone secretion. For example, the pancreas has a major exocrine portion that secretes digestive enzymes and an endocrine portion that secretes hormones. The ovaries and testes secrete hormones and also produce the ova and sperm. Some organs, such as the stomach, intestines, and heart, produce hormones, but their primary function is not hormone secretion.

The endocrine system controls the way your body functions. It produces hormones that travel to all parts of your body to maintain your tissues and organs. Here are a few of the areas governed by the endocrine system:

- Reproduction
- Responses to stress and injury
- Growth and sexual development
- Body energy levels
- Internal balance of body systems
- Bone and muscle strength

When your endocrine glands work together smoothly, your body functions like a choreographed dance, but when something goes awry, your body begins to falter and complain. Because your hormones influence so many different systems of your body, a book such as this one (a "hormone survival guide") requires chapters not only about your reproductive system, but also about your brain and heart and more.

Here are the glands in a woman's endocrine system, in alphabetical order:

- **Adrenal glands.** Your two adrenal glands, which are located on top of your kidneys, release a hormone known as adrenaline when you experience stress. They influence your body's use of energy.
- **Hypothalamus.** Your hypothalamus is an almond-size portion of your brain, located just above the brain stem. It synthesizes and secretes hypothalamic hormones which in turn stimulate your pituitary gland.
- **Ovaries.** These egg-producing organs also produce estrogen and progesterone (hormones about which much of the rest of this book is concerned).
- **Pancreas.** Your pancreas is part of both the endocrine system and the digestive system. It releases insulin, needed by your body to metabolize sugar, as anyone who has struggled with diabetes will know.
- **Parathyroid.** This consists of two pairs of glands that are usually situated behind the thyroid gland. They produce a hormone that, along with

a hormone from the thyroid gland, regulate the calcium content of your blood and bones.

- **Pineal gland.** Located in the center of your brain, resembles a small pine cone (thus "pineal"). It produces several vital hormones, notably melatonin, which influences your sleeping/waking cycles as well as your sexual development.

- **Pituitary gland.** Far down in the alphabetical list but far up the list of importance as endocrine glands go, your pituitary gland drives and guides the rest of your endocrine system and is essential to your growth and maturation, as well as your mental development.

- **Thymus.** Your two-lobed thymus gland can be found between your sternum and your heart. Most active in childhood, it creates T cells for your immune system.

- **Thyroid.** Your thyroid gland is one of the largest endocrine glands in your body, located in the front of your neck near your Adam's apple. The hormones it produces regulate the growth and rate of function of many other systems in your body.

Endocrinologists are medical specialists in hormone function, and they can administer tests to help diagnose hormonal imbalances. They have an ever-increasing comprehension of the complex interactions of human hormones, not only with each other but also with the multitudinous systems and processes within a person's body and environment.

Hormone "balance" is a delicate thing, to be sure. But when your hormones are not working as they should, for whatever reason, you suffer the effects. You may blame your malaise on any number of obvious stress-causing origins, and you may be able to change some of those circumstances, only to fail to address the invisible hormonal imbalances that remain.

Women and Hormones

From the cradle to the grave our hormones play a vitally important role in our health and well-being. As a woman you will be most aware of the operation of the so-called "sex hormones," the estrogens in particular (estradiol, estriol, and estrone).

Women of today are fortunate to have access to much information and choices. Our mothers and grandmothers were not as fortunate, but for the most part their hormonal issues may not have been as severe as the ones we face in this era. This is due in part to the amount of environmental and dietary xenoestrogens to which we are exposed on a daily basis, coming from environmental pollutants, pesticides, plastic-lined cans, stress, and beef, poultry, and milk laden with growth hormones.

Xenoestrogens are substances that exert an estrogen-like effect on our systems, thereby contributing to hormonal imbalance due to estrogen dominance. It is this estrogen dominance that causes early puberty in young girls. When you add in low-ered adrenal function (hypoadrenia) due to high-stress lifestyles and poor diets, com-plete with high caffeine and sugar consumption, you have the makings of a nation of hormonally imbalanced women.

The good news is that whatever your stage of life and sexual maturity, there are ways to regain your hormonal balance and reclaim your edge.

ESTROGEN-PROGESTERONE BALANCE	
Estrogen	Progesterone
Increases body fat	Helps use fat for energy
Increases salt and fluid retention	Acts as a natural diuretic
Increases risk of breast cancer	May help prevent breast cancer
Decreases sex drive	Restores sex drive
Causes headaches and depression	Acts as a natural antidepressant
Impairs blood sugar control	Normalizes blood sugar levels
Increases risk of endometrial cancer	May help prevent endometrial cancer
Reduces oxygen in all cells	Restores proper cell oxygen

PMS

One of a young woman's earliest experiences of hormone fluctuations in her body comes along with puberty—premenstrual syndrome, or PMS. Chapter 4 delves more deeply into the topic, but for now let's sum it up by saying that PMS results from inad-equate levels of progesterone in the second half of the menstrual cycle. This creates an "estrogen dominant" situation. (Estrogen dominance occurs more often in women these days because of xenoestrogens.)

Many women say that they experience most symptoms of PMS in the two-week period before menstruation, when the ratios are widest. In addition, low thyroid, low brain serotonin, poor liver function, and a diet that contains too much salt, caffeine, sugar, and red meat are all implicated in the development of PMS. It has been found that many sufferers have deficiencies in the B vitamins and in minerals. Emotional turmoil and stress can magnify the symptoms. Because of all of the factors that contribute to PMS, there is no one cause and no one treatment. Again, balance is all important.

Premenopause

Premenopause (also known as perimenopause) begins in the average woman around the age of forty and continues until the early fifties when the menstrual period becomes a thing of the past, signaling the beginning of menopause. During this stage of life, many women experience a decrease or even cessation in their progesterone production because of irregular ovarian cycling and ovarian aging. At the same time, estrogen levels may be excessively or moderately high, causing a troubling, continual state of imbalance or estrogen dominance. And therein lies most of the midlife woman's complaints.

Women may experience a plethora of symptoms, some for years on end. These may include fatigue, breast tenderness, foggy thinking, irritability, headaches, insomnia, decreased sex drive, anxiety, depression, allergy symptoms (including asthma), fat gain (especially around the middle), hair loss, mood swings, memory loss, water retention, bone loss, endometrial cancer, breast cancer, slow metabolism, and many others. Hormonal imbalance has far-reaching effects on many tissues in the body, including the heart, brain, blood vessels, bones, uterus, and breasts.

It is possible to smooth premenopause by bringing the levels of estrogen and progesterone back into balance, as long as stress is also well managed. When this is accomplished, women feel wonderful again.

Menopause

With the onset of premenopause and on into the menopausal years (after ovulation and menstrual periods have ceased for good), women experience many of these symptoms:

- Weight gain
- Uterine fibroid tumors
- Sore, lumpy breasts
- Skin that is dry, thinner, wrinkled
- Decreased sex drive
- Painful sexual intercourse
- Irritability, anxiety, possibly depression
- Frequent bladder or vaginal infections
- Achy joints and muscles

- Forgetfulness
- Hot flashes
- Insomnia and interrupted sleep

CHECKLIST FOR HORMONAL/ OVARIAN IMBALANCE

Make note of symptoms or behaviors that occur throughout the month with a frequency or intensity that affects your daily activities or your ability to feel good about yourself.

- ❑ Anxiety
- ❑ Irritability
- ❑ Temporary weight gain
- ❑ Water retention
- ❑ Abdominal bloating
- ❑ Tender/swollen breasts
- ❑ Craving for sweets
- ❑ Heart palpitations
- ❑ Depression
- ❑ Heavy prolonged periods
- ❑ Unusually light periods
- ❑ Irregular periods
- ❑ Bleeding or spotting between periods

Consult your doctor with your concerns. For unusual menstrual bleeding, vaginal sonography (ultrasound) is less invasive than other procedures that might be used to determine whether observation is in order or a more active intervention is called for.

This transitional midlife stage of the menopausal years can be quite a roller-coaster ride—complete with those wild body-temperature fluctuations known as hot flashes.

Hot flashes occur because of fluctuating estrogen levels, which result in increased blood flow to the brain, skin, and organs. This causes a sudden sensation of warmth, usually beginning in the face or chest area and spreading throughout the body. A hot flash may be followed by chills (a "cold flash" of sorts). They can last as long as thirty minutes, although most of them are about two to three minutes long. Sweating and rapid heartbeat are common. As sufferers know all too well, hot flashes can be stimulated by being in a hot environment, and they can be accompanied by an embarrassing reddening of the face, neck, and chest. Because estrogen levels are lowest at night, some women who do not have hot flashes at all during the day nevertheless have a number of them at night. Night hot flashes (or "night sweats") can make restful sleep a thing of the past.

Here's what is happening. At menopause, estrogen production drops by 75 to 90 percent, while progesterone production has virtually stopped. Androgens, the hormones that stimulate the sex drive, drop by 50 percent. Since the appearance of hot flashes coordinates with this hormonal shift, hormones get the blame. In addition, there may be age-related changes in the hypothalamus's control of temperature regulation within the body.

BENEFITS OF ESTROGEN

- Combats dryness generally
- Lowers bad LDL cholesterol
- Has antioxidant effects
- Reduces risk of colon cancer
- Improves skin; reduces wrinkling
- Is neuroprotective of the brain
- Reduces glaucoma
- Influences mood
- Helps prevent urinary urgency and leakage
- Helps maintain vaginal health and comfort
- Maintains bone density

Negative Consequences of Estrogen Dominance

It is those difficult-to-manage symptoms of the middle years' hormonal shifts that drive so many women to seek solutions and relief. Depending on external and internal influences, estrogen will behave well or potentially cause serious damage. While your genes will play a part in how estrogen interacts with your cells, their expression is skewed by many factors. The chance they will give an order for cancer or some other disease process depends to a large extent on multiple dynamics, many of which are under your control.

Since estrogen is broken down in the liver, it makes sense that healthy liver function is important. The liver's role includes "detoxification," which means it takes something that can harm us and changes it into a form that is no longer dangerous. If your liver is working as it should, it can minimize, through detoxification and excretion, production of highly reactive breakdown products of estrogen that can damage DNA and trigger cancer directly or indirectly. Trouble also results when pathogenic gut bacteria in an unbalanced intestine allow estrogen to reenter the circulation. Bad guy bacteria are associated with greater cancer risk, including breast cancer. This threat is increased by a diet high in fat and low in fiber.

Phytoestrogens and other natural nutrients found in a wide variety of plant foods (legumes; clover; fermented, non-GMO soy; kudzu; licorice root) can act as an estrogen or an anti-estrogen, depending on what the body needs. See chapter 14 for more about the hormonal benefits of certain plant foods.

Inherited genetic propensity and obesity each have their own ways of escalating cancer risk. Obesity is a problem because it provides extra fat cells for estrogen production. Getting down to your ideal weight means that you have reduced the territory where estrogen can be made. Additionally, too much insulin in the bloodstream prompts the ovaries to secrete excess testosterone and in turn reduces sex-hormone-binding globulin (SHBG) levels, freeing estrogen to do its damage. The decision to lose weight, if you have added some baby fat to your grown-up frame, is an excellent first choice in any effort made to reduce the chance of having your estrogen misbehave.

CONSUMPTION OF ALCOHOL

For those who decide to drink alcoholic beverages, beware. Estrogen levels are increased with alcohol consumption of more than 12 ounces of beer, 5 ounces of wine, or 1.5 ounces of 80-proof distilled spirits per day.

After taking into account your genes, your prospects for trouble depend significantly on what you eat, how fit and trim you are, and environmental exposure to toxins and exogenous hormones of various types. Numerous pesticides, carcinogens, and certain drugs such as cyclosporine and cimetidine (Tagamet), can cause the metabolite ratio to tilt in favor of developing cancer. This is because so many environmental toxins have structures so similar to estrogen, they can mimic detrimental estrogen metabolites. No matter the source, many are capable of binding to estrogen receptors. Environmental estrogens are known as ecoestrogens or xenoestrogens. (See chapters 2 and 4 for more information.)

Unlike phytoestrogens from food that break down and spend little time in the body, synthetic environmental estrogens linger on the receptors, increasing the potential for harm. Examples include aromatic hydrocarbons and organochlorines found in pesticides, herbicides, plastics, refrigerants, industrial solvents, and many household products.

In addition, there are legitimate concerns about the hormones used to fatten livestock and promote milk production. We know a considerable amount about how these chemicals can alter an animal's life cycle and health. We don't know the full extent of their effect on humans. We must assume that length of exposure, the dose, age, health, and individual genetic diversity make a difference in how much harm is done.

There are so many potential concerns to address. Here are a few of the most common problems women face after the age of forty.

Fatigue

Most women today have a reason to be tired. It is the rare individual whose life is serene and balanced. Instead, women's days are filled with too many stressful demands, which result in shortened and interrupted sleep, along with psychological and spiritual struggles. Medications frequently keep them awake. Physical pain not only makes a person restless, it also increases cortisol and the fight-or-flight response. Does this sound like your experience? If no amount of restorative rest or sleep helps you feel rested—and especially if you are more tired than refreshed thirty minutes after exercising—a deeper problem is likely. Adrenal and thyroid imbalances are apt to be involved and should be addressed.

Especially with women who have lived with much stress or illness, "midlife angst" not readily taken care of by the usual menopause interventions can often be attributed to adrenal problems. The causes are multiple and usually have been years in the making. A genuine effort to live a calmer life is essential for medicinal therapy to work. Restoring adrenal function and rebalancing cortisol may take weeks to months. It took years to compromise adrenal function, and patience is required to undo the damage.

At midlife the adrenals are designed to do double duty and pick up the slack for the ovaries as they begin to shut down their production of sex hormones. If the adrenals are taxed and worn out, they cannot help smooth out the transition into menopause.

This is why many Type-A women experience an almost unbearable menopause, complete with severe anxiety, monster hot flashes, extreme fatigue, and more. These women are often prescribed Paxil, Xanax, and the like just to get them through these transitional years.

Inflammation

Some of the same methods for balancing your hormones also apply to fighting inflammation, because the balance of body chemistry, designed for our good, can be nudged to an imbalance, resulting in harm.

Here is one example of how that imbalance works in your body. Think back to a time when you were out to dinner and food lodged between your teeth. Not wanting to pick your teeth in front of your son's future in-laws, you did some ballet moves with your tongue to dislodge most of whatever was there. You went home and gave your teeth their nightly two-minute scrub, but you were too tired to floss. A tiny speck escaped your probing, and by morning an area of your gum became reddened, swollen, and sore. While you overlooked this minute invader, your body did not. It sent out an arsenal of macrophages (your body's killer cells) and T cells (white blood cells) to annihilate the attacker with a killer dose of chemicals that also set in motion other lifesaving mechanisms. You floss and rinse, and within a day the pain and redness subside. This protective, albeit inflamed, response has been dubbed "friendly fire." Your immune system detected a danger and swiftly responded to minimize damage. It did what it was designed to do.

But as you well know, fire, when not contained, becomes very unfriendly. Inflammatory "fire," when out of control in the body, becomes a major factor in the majority of diseases we encounter as we age. So what is the consequence of deciding not to floss your teeth? You may not develop a sore gum that indicates an invasion of nasty bacteria, but that does not mean you do not have a mini-war going on. Instead of your inflammatory process shutting down and resting until the next true assault, it remains hyped up, but below your awareness, and prepared to act, though it is not clear about why. And act it does. With no invasion to attend to, it begins to attack healthy tissue.

The healthy tissue this harmful inflammation goes after could be within the vessels of the heart. How does this happen? The low-grade infection in your mouth (or infection from some other source) can send out orders to produce more troops (macrophages and T cells), which proceed to attack LDL in your bloodstream, causing it to produce fatty, frothy plaque that digs into artery walls. It stays there, perhaps for years, until immune chemicals, working inside the plaque, literally pop the seal and release blood-clot-producing factors that glom to material in the blood. These factors quickly form clots that sail along until they get stuck in arteries in the neck or brain, causing a stroke, or they block an artery in the heart, resulting in a heart attack. In fact, inflammation is now thought to be the major cause of plaque rupture.

While atherosclerosis is the main cause of plaque development, half of all heart attacks occur in women whose cholesterol levels put them in the safe "atta-girl" category, two-thirds of whom have no major artery blockage. These attacks are caused by overzealous inflammatory processes, so essential for our protection, which become an uncontrolled fire with catastrophic results.

It is understood that inflammation processes are at work with cancer. Lengthy exposure to internal or external toxins or too much sun, among other known cancer-causing agents, appear to switch on the immune system, wherein inflammatory processes, ironically, end up feeding and protecting the rebel cancer cells. Long-term damage from inflammation due to severe heartburn or inflammatory bowel disease increases cancer risk. Arthritis is a known inflammatory disease. It was the discovery that arthritis patients who fought their inflamed joints with anti-inflammatory medication like NSAIDs and aspirin had lowered incidence of Alzheimer's that first tipped scientists to its inflammation connection, as well. Even diabetes is suspect because especially potent proteins involved in inflammation interfere with insulin's ability to regulate blood sugar properly. It is speculated that inflammation may even cause the liver to produce too much blood sugar.

To reduce inflammation as you get older, pay attention to good nutrition for starters. There is no getting around the fact that to maintain inflammatory processes as no more than "friendly fire" requires that you avoid fast food. Eating a high-fat/high-carbohydrate meal will elevate inflammatory processes as long as four hours after your meal. If you stopped at McDonald's for lunch and then at four o'clock had a muffin or doughnut with your friend at the coffee shop, it is possible for inflammatory processes to be elevated for another three or four hours, meaning seven to eight hours of increased chance for damage. The healthier you are, the less damage such a trip to the "wild side" will do. But if you are at risk for heart disease, are diabetic or arthritic, such indulgence could be very risky.

It is interesting to note that exercise actually triggers an increased inflammatory response. But your body, recognizing a good thing when it sees it, immediately sets in motion the production of antioxidants that ultimately reduce the inflammatory response to "friendly fire" levels. Because inflammation involves changes in gastrointestinal function; liver detoxification; and immune, nervous, and endocrine system function, anything that improves overall health, such as exercise, will improve inflammatory processes.

You may have noted a connection between what you eat and increased joint pain. This is because the gastrointestinal tract plays an important role in both local and systemic inflammation. Imbalance of gut bacteria can lead to inflammation throughout your body. Inflammation is lowered when attention is paid to lifestyle, environment, diet, and stress management. Study the chart below to determine how to decrease harmful inflammation processes.

FIGHTING INFLAMMATION

Things That Increase Inflammation	Things That Decrease Inflammation
The wrong fat: omega-6 in corn, safflower, sunflower, and sesame oils	Good fat: omega-3 in olive oil; salmon, walnuts, and flaxseed; raw material for making anti-inflammatory hormones
Fast food; high-fat, low-fiber, processed, contaminated food	Probiotics restore intestinal bacteria balance.
Your own fat cells produce chemicals that direct inflammation processes.	Healthy fat/lean ratio; exercise produces antioxidants, lowers C-reactive protein
Normal LDL plus inflammatory risk factors and high LDL trigger immune system reactions leading to heart attack, stroke, and high blood pressure.	Nitric oxide maintains health of vessel lining, preventing plague formation; exercise, Mediterranean-style diet, statins, ACE inhibitors, beta-blockers, aspirin, lowering blood pressure
Low-grade infections such as gum disease, bronchitis, cold sores, or ulcer-producing bacteria	Soy, exercise, echinacea, adequate rest, reduction of stress, vitamin C to increase immunity
Stress hormones such as cortisol and adrenaline keep immune and inflammatory processes from turning off.	Meditation, prayer, yoga, and massage reduce stress hormones.
Lack of vegetables and fruits	Fruits and vegetables contain phytonutrients, especially antioxidants and flavonoids that block inflammation-promoting hormones, and some (raspberries, raisins, prunes, broccoli, zucchini, green peppers, tomato sauce) may even reduce pain naturally or calm inflammation; bright colors and berries are winners; spices such as turmeric contain the anti-inflammatory curcumin.
Too many high-glycemic foods, processed foods, or fast foods	Whole grains, oatmeal, foods that improve glucose levels
Very high-protein diets	Soy. Genistein/daidzein have anti-inflammatory properties and lower free radicals that cause microscopic damage and inflammation.
Sugary soft drinks	Green or black tea, orange or cranberry juice, red wine
HRT (hormone replacement therapy)	Black cohosh (mild anti-inflammatory)

FIGHTING INFLAMMATION (Cont . . .)	
Things That Increase Inflammation	Things That Decrease Inflammation
Cortisol and NSAID use with gastrointestinal upset	Glucosamine sulfate and chondroitin sulfate; Co-Q$_{10}$; botanicals: oleanolic acid to reduce swelling, rosemary extract (*Rosmarinus officinalis*), turmeric (*Curcuma longa*), boswellia (*Boswellia serrata*), and ginger (*Zingiber officinale*)
Vitamin depletion	Vitamins E, K, and A; carotene, zinc, selenium

When inflammatory (or other) processes go bad and disrupt function by attacking healthy cells, the person is said to have an autoimmune disorder. The body attacks itself. In such cases, T cells fail to make the distinction between "you" and "not you." Women are ten times more likely than men to be afflicted. Seventy-five percent of rheumatoid arthritis sufferers are women, as are 70–80 percent of people with lupus and up to 90 percent with multiple sclerosis. With arthritis, which is the leading cause of disability among adults in the United States, the misguided immune system targets the joints.[3]

Pain is controlled in most cases by anti-inflammatory medications, and in severe cases prednisone or cyclosporine to "turn down" the activity of the immune system, but these drugs have serious side effects.

Surgical Solutions for Hormonally Caused Problems

Some of the most common surgeries in the United States are gynecologic. Many times they are done to relieve a disease process in the uterus itself that is causing troublesome menstrual cycles. Often other means have failed to alleviate the situation, and this is the next option.

Some of the transitional issues in this period of life include changes in the menstrual cycle. Menstrual periods can become longer, heavier, and closer together, with more cramping and clotting. This can be the result of irregular ovulations and poor progesterone levels that do not effectively eliminate the monthly lining of the uterus. Supplementing progesterone through either very low-dose birth control pills or progesterone-only formulations may be all that is needed to regulate the periods. But often there are physical changes in the uterus itself that need surgical correction.

Urinary Tract Infections

Changing ratios of estrogen and progesterone increase the risk of urinary tract infections. In particular, a reduced level of estrogen in a woman's system at midlife tends to enhance the adhesive qualities of the bladder's lining, thereby preventing proper bacterial removal upon urination. In addition, by the time a woman reaches midlife, the muscles of the pelvic floor are weakened as the result of previous pregnancies and deliveries. This can cause the bladder to sag, which in turn contributes to the growth of bacterial colonies. Aging itself, poor posture, spinal disorders, excessive abdominal fat, and chronic constipation are other contributing factors. Most often, however, E. coli bacterium traveling up the urethra is the culprit. If bladder infections are ignored due to hectic lifestyles and not addressed quickly, the kidneys can be infected as well, making it a much more serious condition that can lead to kidney failure.

Bladder infection symptoms include painful, frequent, and urgent urination with pain in the lower back and abdomen, chills, and fever as the body tries to fight the infection. The urine is often cloudy with a strong smell. Occasionally traces of blood are seen. It is essential to begin attacking the infection at the first sign of discomfort.

Normal Passage of Life

It isn't only symptoms of hormonal imbalance that are bothering many midlife women. Many are also out of touch with their bodies and their feelings. Some have lost touch socially as they try to balance work and family life. They do not nurture themselves and wind up tired, bewildered, anxious, and depressed.

It is unfortunate that many in the medical profession have tended to treat this phase of life as a disease state rather than a normal passage of life. In years past women with these same symptoms were nurtured with herbs, reassurance, and time-tested wisdom from older women who had taken the journey before them. Today's lifestyles are even more hectic, and stress levels are relentlessly high, further driving hormone levels down.

Many in the medical profession have tried to deal with these negative symptoms that occur at midlife with prescription medications that elevate mood and alter the personality. Synthetic hormone replacement has been a standard of midlife care. In 2002 a landmark US National Institutes of Health study, the Woman's Health Initiative (WHI), was halted abruptly when it was found that Prempro, a synthetic estrogen/progestin medication, actually increased a women's risk of heart attack, stroke, and breast cancer.[4] The study was aborted due to the possibility of endangering the lives of the women in the study. As a result, for the first time in several decades both doctors and patients started rethinking midlife hormonal health. Now research had shown that excess estrogen is a dangerous cancer-promoter. It fuels endometrial growth (endometriosis), encourages fibroid growth, contributes to fibrocystic breasts, and causes weight gain, headaches, gallbladder problems, and heavier periods, just to name a few of the negatives.

GET MOVING

Just thirty minutes of moderate activity most days, which can be done in smaller increments, dilates blood vessels, decreases resistance to blood flow, enhances HDL/LDL ratio, conditions the heart to pump more efficiently, reduces body fat, burns excess sugar, makes cells more sensitive to insulin, increases energy and fights depression, Alzheimer's, and osteoporosis.

Each individual woman is different. Many factors influence the timing of premenopause and menopause, including trauma, surgery, and low body weight, which brings on early menopause due to decreased hormone output by the ovaries. Anorexia can cause the ovaries to shut down completely. Being overweight can delay menopause because extra fat increases estradiol. Physically active and well-nourished women experience late menopause while smokers experience earlier menopause. Adrenal exhaustion from too much stress and poor diet can cause early menopause.

As complex as it is to contemplate this season of life, there are many simple things you can do to make it more balanced. For advice on specific topics, you can start by reading the pertinent chapters of this book.

Chapter 3

THEY MEANT WELL

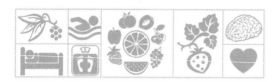

BEFORE THE EARLY 1900s most women lived only to the age of forty-seven or forty-eight, so menopause was comparatively rare. Women simply didn't live long enough to go through it! But as women's life spans began to increase, doctors began seeing certain symptoms appearing in aging women: hot flashes, mood swings, depression, anxiety, and sleeplessness. Unfortunately these symptoms were grossly misunderstood by the medical community.

When a woman who was sitting in a perfectly cool room suddenly broke out into a sweat, or when she sobbed uncontrollably for days at a time, doctors diagnosed it as the only thing they understood it to be: insanity. Many menopausal women were admitted to psychiatric hospitals simply for displaying what we now consider normal symptoms that greet women as they grow older.

In the early 1800s a French physician had codified this belief in his book, *De la Menopause ou de l'Âge Critique des Femmes*.[1] If a woman was fortunate to live long enough to reach menopause, he wrote, she would be unfortunate enough to have to face a laundry list of problems accompanied by mental deterioration. Picking up the theme, a British physician wrote in 1887 that "uterine" disease was a factor in insanity.[2] Sensing ovarian demise, he observed, ovaries at midlife send out signals that caused, if not insanity, then "extreme nervousness."[3] Even as recently as the late 1960s, medical schools taught about a psychological disorder of midlife women called "involutional melancholia."

Hormones Enter the Scene

Then in the 1930s hormones came to the attention of physicians, although it wasn't until the 1960s that replenishing them at midlife became the treatment of choice. Doctors began to understand that menopausal symptoms were caused by the body's ceasing to produce the hormone estrogen.

The most widely used estrogen supplement, Premarin, was approved in 1942. Premarin since became the most common estrogen hormone prescription written in America. Premarin contains estrogens that are derived from the urine of pregnant mares. Its acceptance by the Food and Drug Administration (FDA) was based on satisfactory chemistry and manufacturing plus reports from clinical trials that the drug was safe for its intended use, which was defined as treatment of menopausal symptoms and related conditions. It did work. Amazingly the hot flashes, the night sweats, and the mood swings all disappeared.

But then a startling problem began to take place: uterine cancer rates began to skyrocket. Some statistics even show a leap of 13 to 15 percent among women who took prescription estrogen. Eventually doctors discovered that adding progestin to the estrogen that women were taking helped protect the uterine lining and decrease the risk of uterine cancer. But then the risk of breast cancer seemed to leap sky high.

Now it is important to stress that most doctors are motivated by the desire to help people, but they will be the first to admit that they are limited in what they understand and in their ability to help. So it is true that many women have suffered at their hands. When the medical treatments that cured hot flashes turned out to cause cancer; it was time to seek out a better way.

COMMON ASSUMPTIONS ABOUT HORMONE REPLACEMENT

Challenge your own assumptions. Ask yourself, "Why do I assume this?"

- If I am menopausal, then I have to do something.
- If pharmaceutical hormones (HRT) are the problem, then natural hormones (nature-identical hormones) are the answer.
- If I feel better on HRT, then I can stay on it, as long as I cut down on how much I use.
- If I don't want to or no longer feel I can use hormone therapy, then I will protect myself by buying all natural products from the health food store.
- If hormones cause serious health problems, then I should never take them.
- If hormones cause breast cancer, then I have cancer because I took them.

In the 1990s a number of books were written that unbolted the door to an open discussion of menopause. While the perception of menopause as disease was beginning to be challenged, most conversations still focused on the misery and disruption of the transition. Writings about women becoming independent, rearranging their lives, and being happy were chiefly found among more fringe audiences. Neither being sick nor being wizened is particularly appealing to anybody.

Physicians obligingly wrote forty-six million prescriptions for the hormone Premarin in its various formulations in the year 2000.[4] With more than one billion sales in the United States, it was the second most frequently prescribed medication. Now it has been the leading hormonal choice of the medical profession for over fifty years. Premarin has weathered protests of the treatment of pregnant mares from which it is derived. It has survived the fact that a full 40 percent of women never filled their prescription for hormones and that more than half discontinued use within a year.

The introduction of Premarin had predated the current requirements for comprehensive analysis of every component in any product under review. No one at the time knew everything it contained, and therefore, testing what each component did was not possible. The thinking of the day was that most estrogens could be judged by their final potency and that everything in them worked to that end. The other hormone commonly prescribed with Premarin is Provera. Provera is a synthetic form of progesterone that is commonly taken in conjunction with Premarin in order to prevent cancer of the uterus.

Today researchers know that not all estrogens or progestogens work the same way, and therefore may not be interchangeable. Even the method of delivery (in what form you take them) makes a difference.

It is interesting to note that in 1997 a generic form of Premarin was turned down by the FDA because all the ingredients and their exact mechanism of action had still not been defined and therefore could not be duplicated. In 1990 Wyeth, the company that produces Premarin, petitioned the FDA for new labeling that went beyond relief of menopausal symptoms to include cardiovascular protection. The FDA asked for proof, so Wyeth initiated a well-designed double-blind, randomized, placebo-controlled clinical trial, the Heart and Estrogen/Progestin Replacement Study (HERS).[5]

To everyone's dismay, no significant overall difference in the occurrence of cardiovascular disease was noted, despite 10 to 11 percent drops in low-density lipoprotein (LDL—the bad cholesterol) and equivalent increases in HDL (the good cholesterol). This was the complete opposite of the conventional wisdom of the medical profession. The follow-up HERS II study was designed to determine if hormone replacement therapy (HRT) provided cardiovascular protection for older women who already suffered from heart disease. The unexpected conclusion was that such women were at increased risk, especially if they were just starting an HRT regimen.

Subsequent analysis of data from the HERS study found that women on estrogen and progestin with no urinary incontinence at baseline (average age, sixty-six, eighteen years past menopause) found a twofold increase in urge incontinence and fourfold increase in stress incontinence, and the risk of developing the disorders increased with time.[6]

The black eye that HRT received from the two HERS studies was nothing compared to the knockout punch of the Women's Health Initiative study termination in July of 2002. The *Journal of the American Medical Association* (*JAMA*) reported that the Women's Health Initiative (WHI), a study of 161,809 postmenopausal women (fifty to seventy-nine years old) was canceled—at least a portion of it. The women had been placed on estrogen/progestin, or estrogen only, and monitored for coronary heart disease, venous thrombotic events, breast cancer, colon cancer, and fractures. When a predetermined "global index" that measures when risk outweighs benefit reached the critical point, the estrogen/progestin arm of the study was discontinued.

Simply stated, analysis of all the information revealed that for every ten thousand women receiving estrogen/progestin HRT (Prempro or Premphase), there would be eight more breast cancers, eight more strokes, seven more heart attacks, eighteen more venous-thrombotic events, as well as six fewer colon cancers and five fewer hip fractures than among women not receiving HRT.[7] Combination hormone replacement therapy did not convey the unconditional health benefits as previously accepted by the medical community. Even though Premarin and Provera seem to help to prevent uterine cancer, they do not prevent breast or ovarian cancer. In fact, estrogen actually fuels these cancers. In addition, these synthetic hormones cause water retention and excessive accumulation of fat, especially in the abdomen, hips, thighs, and breasts. There was an immediate drop in prescriptions by 40 percent—and that was just the beginning.

The alarming WHI results do not apply to every conceivable combination and type of hormone replacement. The outcome pertains to the estrogen Premarin and the progestin Provera. But realistically other choices, nature-identical or synthetic, have not yet been proven to be better and safer.

Since the publication of the WHI study, two other smaller analyses have conveyed the same dismal results for heart protection. When considering this preponderance of evidence, it is clear that women who are on HRT to prevent heart disease should stop. Those solely on HRT for osteoporosis risk or disease should, with their physicians, consider discontinuing its use. Young women with premature menopause and/or those who have had hysterectomies, however, are advised to continue its use. Recommendations may change, so it is wise to keep in touch with your doctor and to check the National Institute of Health (NIH) website periodically.

WOMEN'S HEALTH INITIATIVE STUDY OUTCOMES[8]		
Outcomes	Hazard Ratio	Increased Risk In 10,000 Women Taking Prempro for One Year
Coronary heart disease (CHD)	+29 percent	7 more CHD events
Stroke	+41 percent	8 more strokes
Venous thromboembolism/ blood clots (VTE)	+111 percent	18 more VTEs
Breast cancer	+26 percent	8 more invasive breast cancers
Hip fracture	-37 percent	5 fewer hip fractures

How did it happen that a drug regimen was so universally accepted when no previous controlled trials had ever shown definitively that HRT prevented cardiovascular disease, stroke, Alzheimer's, or even wrinkles? This is an interesting question when contemplated in the context of the medical community's almost universal cry against the use of botanicals and supplements for lack of proof as measured by double-blind, placebo-controlled studies (ignoring two thousand years of effective and safe use of many natural products). Doctors had become believers in HRT without proof of its efficacy. And women cannot be absolved of their role. The promise and hope of "feminine forever," "youthful evermore," a "pill for an ill" are strong motivations to beat a hasty path to the nearest doctor's office. We see the same behavior with allergy medicines, acid reflux treatments, and weight-loss preparations. Prompted by the mix of science and advertising on television, it's the direct-to-consumer appeal, served alongside our morning coffee, that results in demands for prescriptions.

> Menopause as a natural, physical life transition has symptoms of hot flashes that occur in up to 80 percent of women. However, physicians treat menopause as a disease.

That said, clearly the greatest influence came about because the drug companies told physicians that HRT was a good thing. You may be unaware that drug companies are responsible for much of the post-medical-school-education a physician receives. With the overwhelming task of keeping up on the latest technology and product developments, it is natural for doctors to seek the bottom line, the summary version. But this can be a dangerous practice. Researchers funded by the drug company, for instance, had given presentations at conferences that reinterpreted the HERS study to say there was benefit from HRT over time, ignoring that cumulative cardiovascular events were similar between the treated and control groups. The new logic went so far as to state that because some women had suffered earlier cardiovascular events, they would be saved by HRT from having more of them later, and that if they got breast cancer, it would be less deadly if they had taken HRT. They insisted that those in HERS II who already had cardiovascular disease were simply too sick to get the benefit, while women who were healthy would be helped by HRT.

> **Q:** How do I go off hormone replacement?
> **A:** There is no reason you cannot simply stop taking hormones. You will not suffer any untoward medical consequence. In fact, there are many women who cannot tell the difference from one day to the next. That said, other women will undoubtedly suffer through some uncomfortable symptoms—that will prove bearable—and the deed is done. For those whose symptoms measure on the Richter scale, it is wise to abandon the "grin-and-bear-it" approach and go back on hormones and taper off gradually. It is probably wiser (and from a natural medicine perspective, easier on your body) to taper off. If you are on the highest dose of estrogen (0.625 mg), you could cut your pills in two or ask your physician for a prescription for a lower dose (0.3 mg). Should you be fearful of symptoms being more than you can bear, try alternating days (0.625 with 0.3 mg) for a month, working toward the lower dose only and tapering off from there. The same "tapering" can be used with the "patch," which can be cut in two. Most women simply extend their time between pills until they feel comfortable enough to stop completely.

The numerous studies demonstrating that women who took estrogen had fewer cardiovascular events is likely explained by what some researchers suspected all along: HRT users have been shown to have fewer health risks in the first place, because they are more likely to take care of themselves. Apparently HRT can serve as a marker for less heart disease, but not as a player in its reduction.[9]

The withdrawal of HRT as the main "fix" for "women of a certain age" created a plethora of "What Now?" articles in medical and lay journals, and some articles in professional journals didn't sound much more hopeful than those from the 1800s. The

[handwritten annotation at top: science-based wellness that assess + treats underlying cause of illness thro individualise tailored therapies to reske health + improve functs]

fallout from the WHI study had become a defining moment for gynecologists. Lower doses? New methods of delivery? Different formulations? Return to straight estrogen? Only some have pursued a serious discussion of botanicals and of improving overall health as a means of reducing menopause symptomology.

The Problem With Standard Treatments

Back to the fundamental problem—the fact that too often doctors treat menopause as a disease instead of a natural life transition. The conventional wisdom that women need medicinal hormones at menopause implies a number of notions about aging. Assumptions such as, "*If* menopause is a disease, *then* all women who stop making estrogen in the amounts they did as young women are going to become ill very soon after they stop menstruating and will get sick and die at a relatively young age as compared to men."

Is this true? No. Women do not die when they are no longer able to reproduce. Closer scrutiny, a reality check, if you will, reveals:

1. Women, on average, outlive men.

2. Hormones don't disappear completely; they decline gradually and continue to support bone, heart health, and other vital functions.

3. There appears to be an adaptive advantage to socializing humans when several generations are involved. Mature adults possessing wisdom and insight most profoundly influence the young when the business and distraction of childbearing and child-rearing come to an end.

Declining hormones are simply a part of aging, but not a death sentence.

If menopause were truly a disease, then needing a pill to fix it would be a logical conclusion. But popping a pill at midlife won't result in healthy aging, a healthy menopause, and a balanced life. It makes no difference how dramatic the outcomes in the short run, ultimately all pills are a temporary fix if they are not addressing the underlying cause of the problem at hand. Whether you use herbs, vitamins, minerals, biofeedback, acupuncture, massage, chiropractic, osteopathy, Ayurveda, or Chinese medicine, if you treat the symptom and not the cause, the outcome will always be disappointing.

Functional Medicine

Functional medicine is a science-based health care approach that assesses and treats underlying causes of illness through individually tailored therapies to restore health and improve function. It differs from alternative approaches that depend more on the integration of spiritual, ritual, and empirical (gained from observation or experience) medical knowledge. And functional medicine differs from the "allopathic" approach (conventional medicine), that emphasizes diagnosis of disease, followed by application of a standard treatment that is most likely to apply to a majority of patients.

A functional medicine practitioner believes that prompt intervention will prevent a progression of illness that can become unbearable emotionally, spiritually, financially, and physically. He or she practices a type of "upstream" (studying root or underlying causes) medicine by interrupting chemical processes that could leave a person sick "downstream." Regulating blood pressure is an example; using biochemistry, physiology, nutrition, and psychosocial considerations to understand and improve a person's physiological, emotional, cognitive, and physical functioning, a functional medicine professional doesn't assume that the high blood pressure a patient has is the result of the same metabolic defect in a long range of physiological actions that is universal for everyone. Similar symptoms can result from different metabolic alterations, and so addressing the "system" will be a better approach than intervention at one step along the way. And if someone is already chronically ill, secondary preventative and therapeutic interventions will be recommended. By contrast, a conventional physician will most likely suggest a pill that will effectively work to bring blood pressure down, but nothing will likely be done about the underlying causes.

Anything that assists and augments the body's natural design and the healing processes simply makes sense. The body is not a series of isolated parts but an integrated whole. The goal is to heal without creating further harm. A functional practitioner is far less apt to apply a "wait-and-see" approach to standard treatments, because he or she believes that even small imbalances can make a difference in long-term health. Suboptimal health is a significant factor in the development and experience of chronic illness and degenerative diseases.

For the functional doctor, the specifics of how and when to intervene are not based solely on accepted evidence as defined in a textbook or observed in a laboratory result. Treatment is not determined by an arbitrary cutoff point but through a "functional" assessment of how efficiently and effectively the body, or a specific cell, organ, or system in the body, is working. The goal in a functional approach is to find root causes and suggest interventions that work long-term. In essence, the bottom line is that we are not robots programmed to perform physiologically or spiritually like everyone else in a rigid, unchangeable way. The particulars of our unique functions may require some detective work, but these things are not undecipherable.

If you want to pursue the possibility of treatment by a functional doctor, there are various ways to do so. There is a training center for physicians who would like to brush up on their functional medicine skills, The Institute for Functional Medicine (a nonprofit educational organization: www.functionalmedicine.org). Contacting them is a good first start for a referral in your area. You are also apt to find knowledgeable practitioners among doctors of osteopathy (DO), whose philosophy has always been to seek ways the body might heal itself. Many times physician assistants (PA), nurse practitioners (NP), and/or registered dieticians (RD) specializing in women's health are knowledgeable or at least open to becoming a health partner.

Any health practitioner who listens, respects your input, considers your emotional and physical environment and metabolic balance, and is sensitive to your biochemical individuality is a "keeper." Functional medicine necessitates taking a balanced approach to treatment. Such a practitioner must be willing to refer or to order potent medicines and drastic, lifesaving procedures when necessary—without allowing attention to preventative, chronic, and degenerative health to be squeezed out.

What Can You Do?

Was HRT ever really necessary? Its use can be compared to getting fitted for a pair of glasses. You go to the ophthalmologist because you have a problem seeing; otherwise you would not choose to be fitted for glasses. You go to the gynecologist for HRT because you have a verifiable problem with hormone imbalance that requires hormones. Or, as is true for the majority, you go because of the prevailing belief that just being menopausal makes them essential. If you lose your glasses and cannot find someone to evaluate your eyesight and fit you for a better pair of glasses, you learn to live with your "new" vision. Your body's other senses are refined to compensate for diminished sight. Taste, touch, smell, and hearing come to your rescue—automatically. Your world is interpreted through a "lens" not dominated by sight alone.

If you lose your hormone replacement therapy, in the same way, your body compensates—by adjusting to a gradual decline. Lower hormone levels are normal as we age, just as declining eyesight, hearing, and the senses of touch, taste, and smell are. However, there is a big difference between the ways we improve our senses—with glasses, hearing aids, special diets, supplements, and specialized eye exercises—and the way we improve our hormonal balance. These "sense" remedies have no downside; the risk to benefit ratio is in favor of benefit. However, trying to remedy hormonal decline with HRT or in other ways has a risk factor that must be considered.

Adding hormones and wearing glasses are solutions to real problems of impaired function, but they are like comparing apples and oranges because one (wearing glasses) has little or no risk factor, and the other (HRT) does. For sake of the analogy, your body adjusts to lowered hormones as it does to seeing without your glasses. This adjustment does not mean you are settling for less; it simply means you have the opportunity to explore, experience, and explain reality with a different perspective than you had when you were living in a twenty-year-old hormonally charged body.

It is important to understand how we got to a place where we believed that estrogen was a silver bullet. Unless you suffered from a clinical imbalance, the truth about hormones is that you more than likely never needed additional hormones at menopause in the first place. How did we all come to believe hormones at midlife were essential? Even the alternative medical community cast their vote for hormones—as long as they were "natural." The question to ponder is, "Who persuaded women they were sick and needed medicinal hormones?"

If you are menopausal and you have not first tried controlling hot flashes and vaginal distress naturally, you should do so before starting HRT. In this way, it may be possible for the majority who are unable to relieve symptoms naturally to use HRT for a very short period of time to manage hot flashes only when they are at their worst. Hot flashes do not last forever (although they may seem to!), and women should avoid or try to wean themselves off HRT as soon as possible. At present, there is no long-term evidence that pharmaceutically derived substitutes for estrogen (phytoestrogens from soy and other plant sources that act as selective estrogen receptor modulators) are safer than HRT. (See below for more about phytoestrogens.)

> **Q:** Is there a safe length of time for taking HRT?
> **A:** The general consensus is that should you decide to use HRT for symptom relief (hot flashes and vaginal dryness only), or you are already taking it, it ought to be continued for the shortest time possible. Sophisticated diagnostic tests may eventually delineate risk of HRT for every individual. Since risk increases with each additional year of use, an effort to taper off every six months is advised. Basically, with a few individual exceptions, no responsible medical practitioner (or their professional organization) is recommending hormone use for longer than three to five years.

Should you decide to use HRT, select the lowest effective dose. You might consider transdermal (patch) estrogen to reduce the production of harmful metabolites. Persons with gallstones or a poorly functioning liver or digestive tract should certainly give this consideration. Women who have problems with vaginal dryness and urinary control are estrogen-deprived. The vulva, vagina, urethra, bladder neck, and bladder are rich in estrogen receptors and responsive to local hormonal therapy. The problem is progressive, and when treatment is stopped, it is almost always likely to return. This means that if you happen to be a woman who has been unable to resolve what is known medically as "urogenital atrophy" with natural solutions, you may find that regular application of a hormone directly into the vagina is essential. After an initial "loading" dose, creams or tablets used one to three times a week are enough to maintain vaginal health, which is achieved usually within a month or in severe cases within six months. The dosage is low and little hormone is absorbed into the bloodstream. Maintaining the thickness of the vaginal walls contributes to keeping the hormones localized—a good reason for not letting urogenital atrophy get out of hand. Nonhormonal moisturizers and water-soluble lubricants decrease pain and irritation but do not fix the underlying cause. Do not be embarrassed to bring this problem to the attention of your physician. Do note, however, that urinary incontinence can have other causes such as weight, number of children, diabetes, or smoking.

Ever since women have been able to control fertility, get a good education, and become more active and healthy, they have also, as the biggest users of health care, had considerable influence in its direction. It is the aging of the baby boomers that is the stimulus for antiaging products. It is to be hoped that their passion will embrace more than the futility of chasing youth. Healthy aging is a far more realistic, attainable, and worthwhile goal.

While awareness of the power of lifestyle to influence health without serious side effects is increasing, for many physicians, their practice of healing remains centered on medical technology and pharmaceuticals. As yet, training has not caught up with the new understanding of the enormous value and safety of nutrition, natural supplementation, exercise, and healthy lifestyle practices in disease prevention and treatment.

Plant-Derived Phytoestrogens

In pursuit of relief from menopausal miseries, many women have turned to plant-derived phytoestrogens such as diosgenin, a natural progesterone that is usually derived either from soybeans or tropical wild yams. (Note that fermented, non-GMO, and organic soy foods such as tempeh, miso, natto, soy sauce, and tofu are recommended over processed soy protein products such as milk, cheese, and meat substitutes. Note also that many products that claim to have wild yam extract may not contain any progesterone.) Natural progesterone found in phytoestrogens can help to alleviate depression. It has a calming effect on the brain. Women who are experiencing hot flashes can take natural progesterone cream with approximately 480 milligrams of progesterone per ounce, which can be found at health food stores. They can use one-quarter teaspoon of natural progesterone cream twice a day (approximately 20 milligrams a day), rubbing the cream on the neck, upper chest, breasts, inner arms, palms, and thighs, rotating the sites daily. Those who take natural progesterone capsules orally must take a much larger dose, since the liver will eliminate a large part of the supplement almost immediately.

If natural progesterone fails to control the symptoms of menopause, and especially if a woman is prone to osteoporosis and has a family history of osteoporosis, natural estrogen can be used as a supplement. The most commonly recommended natural estrogen preparations are triple estrogen or biestrogen. Triple estrogen is 80 percent estriol, 10 percent estradiol, and 10 percent estrone. Biestrogen is 90 percent estriol and 10 estradiol. Estriol is the safest form of estrogen with the fewest side effects. Estradiol is a thousand times more potent than estriol in stimulating the breast tissue. Estriol is, therefore, much safer to use than estradiol. A woman can use triple estrogen in cream form, as in natural progesterone cream, or in capsule form.

Applying natural estriol cream intra-vaginally can combat dryness and help prevent vaginal and bladder infections. This cream requires a physician's prescription and must be obtained from a compounding pharmacy.

Forget About a Silver Bullet

Despite the varied opinions, when it comes right down to it, most women really don't know what to do. Especially disconcerting is the discovery that their doctors appear not to know either! After all, at their 2001 checkup they were told that if they refused to take hormones, they could plan on becoming the proverbial dried-up prune, humped over with osteoporosis, and poised for a heart attack followed by a stroke. The only "good" news was that the decision not to take hormones would result also in loss of memory, so at least they wouldn't be aware of how bad off they were! The 2002 checkup found many of those same doctors doing an about-face. HRT in one year had gone from a woman's salvation to a cancer-causing, stroke-producing trauma waiting to happen. It is a surprise that "whiplash" has not been added to the list of problems with hormones!

The change of heart over hormones is not the only news that has undermined public confidence in the medical profession's recommendations. Controversy exists over the validity of regular mammograms, high-fiber diets, and vitamin E for heart disease. Knee surgery for osteoarthritis has been labeled ineffective. The new Cox-2 inhibitors and Vioxx advertised as "kinder, gentler" medications for arthritis have been found to cause ulcers just like the previous less-expensive versions. The government's food pyramid makes no sense to anyone, and, horror of horrors, just when you learn to cook a totally new way, you are told you need fat in your diet after all. In whom and in what is a woman to put her faith?

It is clear that complete dependence on medical authority is not the choice. It never has been. Complete dependence on any authority is not a good idea. The pressure to surrender power to specialists in every field is a likely explanation and one of the major reasons why so many of us feel helpless. Doctors were never the clairvoyants we fantasized them to be. While some physicians may have reveled in such authority, most were painfully aware of the shortcomings of attempting to make a patient well without his or her participation and cooperation. Demanding that our physicians do for us what we were supposed to do ourselves makes wellness an illusory dream.

If physicians can't do it for us, can technology? This is the age of technology, after all. Search long enough on the Internet, and answers will be found. Or will they? Apparently most people missed class the day the teacher defined science as a means of discovery, not the source of definitive answers, especially answers about health.

Still, our hope lies firmly rooted in the belief that quick fixes exist and that a wonder pill is out there to keep us in-line skating into our seventh decade, acing the *New York Times* crossword puzzle, melting off those extra pounds, and forever banishing hot flashes. All we need to do, we daydream, is pick the miraculous formulary off the shelves of our local pharmacy.

That a quick fix might not exist is particularly rejected by baby boomers. They have no intention of contending with problems of aging. If the infamous "silver bullet" is not out there at the moment, it will be soon (or so they think)—just stay tuned.

Realistically, what if there is no silver bullet? What if prevention and healing are equally important, and there are no guarantees of feeling no pain? When our Creator designed the human body as male and female, He declared this complex and brilliant system to be "very good" (Gen. 1:31). The magic and mystery of health lies not in the design of a miracle pill, but in the design itself.

Good hormonal health involves restoring a perfect, age-appropriate design.

Chapter 4

REGULATING PMS SYMPTOMS AND MENSTRUAL CYCLES

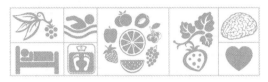

A WOMAN'S BODY IS far more complex and more wonderful than any machine ever made. At birth a baby girl has about seven hundred thousand eggs in her ovaries. By the time she reaches puberty, many of these eggs dissolve, leaving only four hundred thousand. Even so, this young woman will experience only about four hundred to five hundred ovulations in her lifetime when an egg is actually released from an ovary.

The hormone estrogen is only one of many hormones involved in this incredible process. When a young girl begins her monthly menstrual cycle, her body begins releasing and orchestrating an intricate symphony of many different powerful hormones. These hormones are the catalyst for everything that takes place.

The Cycle

The hypothalamus, the pituitary gland, and the ovaries release these powerful hormones. The hormone GnRH (gonadotropin-releasing hormone) triggers the release of hormones from the pituitary gland. GnRH then triggers the pituitary gland to secrete two hormones that cause the egg to mature and eventually to be released from the ovaries.

On average the menstrual cycle is twenty-eight days, with some women bleeding for only three to four days, while others experiencing five to seven days of menstrual flow. The menstrual cycle is divided into three phases. The first stage is marked by the first day of bleeding (referred to as Day 1 of the menstrual cycle) when the woman's body sheds blood and the endometrium (or lining of the uterus). Many women will develop problems with this stage, such as dysmenorrhea (painful periods) and/or menorrhagia (heavy periods).

The second stage of the menstrual cycle is the follicular/proliferative phase. The ovary produces estrogen, and the increasing amounts of estrogen cause the endometrium to grow and reach its maximal thickness at the time of ovulation. Shortly after a woman starts her period, the pituitary gland begins to release FSH (follicle-stimulating hormone). FSH stimulates the growth of about six to twelve eggs and their sacs, called follicles, in the ovaries. Only one egg will fully mature and be released from the ovary. The other eggs and their sacs will then dissolve.

About day fourteen of the menstrual cycle, which is usually right in the middle, marks the beginning of the third stage of the menstrual cycle, the luteal/secretory stage. The pituitary gland releases another hormone called LH (luteinizing hormone) in the brain. This hormone causes the follicle to swell and rupture, releasing the egg from the ovary, which is called ovulation. Some women can actually feel a twinge of pain in one side or the other when they ovulate.

Prior to the release of the egg, estrogen levels increase. Estrogen causes the lining of the uterus to thicken to prepare to receive the egg.

After the ruptured follicle has released its egg, the cells lining the ruptured follicle form the corpus luteum, which secretes the hormone progesterone. This progesterone signals the lining of the uterus to thicken even more, causing the endometrium to convert from a proliferative to a secretory state. As estrogen and other related hormone levels rise, a signal is then sent to the pituitary gland to stop producing LH and FSH. When these hormones decrease, the corpus luteum begins to degenerate, which signals a drop of both estrogen and progesterone. When these two hormone levels drop, the lining of the uterus sloughs off and menstruation begins.

This is not the end, however. The symphony plays on as the pituitary gland once again begins to secrete FSH and LH, which again stimulates more follicles to be developed. Now the entire cycle begins all over again.

Interplay of Hormones

This intricate interplay of hormones within the menstrual cycle is properly orchestrated by three players: the hypothalamus, the pituitary gland, and the ovaries. It's vital that these players produce and secrete the necessary hormones at just the right time in the woman's cycle. This delicate balance of hormones can be upset by many different factors.

All steroid hormones, which include progesterone and estrogen, are first manufactured from cholesterol. Cholesterol, as everyone knows, comes from what a person eats. We have learned that cholesterol is the enemy—but it actually forms the foundation of all steroid sex hormones. Therefore, a small amount of cholesterol or saturated fat in the diet is necessary for hormonal balance.

Cholesterol is converted to pregnenolone, which is eventually converted to progesterone and estrogen. Many steps take place along the way. But if the body lacks the raw materials for this process, it can't make sufficient amounts of hormones. Without enough of the right ingredients, the outcome will doubtless be affected—and the body's delicate hormonal balance will be thrown off.

Those raw materials include cholesterol, specific vitamins, minerals, and enzymes—especially magnesium and vitamin B. Too much stress can also throw off hormonal balance as well. Stress causes excessive amounts of cortisol to be released into the bloodstream. As cortisol levels rise, the body will begin to demand more and more progesterone. That's because cortisol is actually made from progesterone. This also leads to symptoms of PMS.

FACTS ABOUT INFERTILITY

About 10 percent of women (6.1 million) in the United States ages fifteen to forty-four have difficulty getting pregnant or carrying a baby, according to the National Center for Health Statistics of the Centers for Disease Control and Prevention. In the United States about 20 percent of women have their first child after age thirty-five. But one-third of such couples have fertility problems.[1]

The Estrogen and Progesterone Dance

Let's take a closer look at each of these powerful hormones and why they are so important to a woman's health.

Estrogen

People are sometimes surprised to learn there is more than one type of estrogen. Actually, including plant-made estrogens and man-made varieties, there are several:

- Estradiol, which is produced in the ovaries
- Estrone, which is produced in fatty tissues
- Estriol, which is produced primarily in the adrenal glands
- Xenoestrogens, which are environmental chemicals that work like estrogens in a woman's body
- Phytoestrogens, which are plant compounds with weak, estrogen-like effects
- Synthetic estrogen, which is used in hormone replacement therapy and birth control pills

In a manner of speaking, estrogen is actually what makes a girl a woman. This mighty hormone is the key that unlocks a little girl's development of sexual characteristics, including the breasts, pubic hair, and female sex organs. Estrogen is also critical in pregnancy and in maintaining the menstrual cycle. It stimulates the lining of the uterus to grow, preparing a woman's body for pregnancy.

Estrogen stimulates cell growth, and too much estrogen can actually be a promoter for cancer of the breast, uterus, and ovaries. That's where progesterone comes in. Progesterone helps to prevent cancer by balancing the hormones and minimizing the growth properties of estrogen.

Estrogen dominance

The concept of "estrogen dominance" was brought to light by the physician Dr. John Lee, influenced by the prior research of Dr. Raymond Peat. Estrogen dominance is simply estrogen that has not been balanced by progesterone. Rather than blaming the lack of progesterone outright for menopausal symptoms, we can view it more in terms of lack of balance.

Estrogen dominance exacerbates PMS symptoms during the ten to twenty years before menopause (premenopause), usually when a woman is between ages thirty and fifty. Common symptoms include those of PMS: weight gain, fatigue, irritability, mood swings and depression, tender (and enlarged or lumpy) breasts, uterine fibroid tumors, endometriosis, migraine headaches, forgetfulness, problems conceiving, cold hands and feet, and menstrual irregularities such as bleeding between periods, very light periods, or very heavy periods.

Common causes of estrogen dominance include:

- Too much stress
- Hysterectomy
- Tubal ligation
- Some birth control pills
- Going through premenopause when the body continues to secrete estrogen but its level of progesterone is significantly depleted because of not ovulating
- A poorly functioning liver
- Drinking too much alcohol
- Excessive use of prescription medications
- Excessive use of over-the-counter medications such as Tylenol that can place a strain on the liver

Other contributors to estrogen dominance include the proliferation of xenoestrogens and agricultural additives.

Xenoestrogens.

Xeno is Greek for alien, or stranger. Estrogen dominance can be caused by xeno-hormones, or xenoestrogens, which are man-made chemicals in the environment that fool the body into believing they are natural estrogen. The bloodstream invites these strangers in, just like a Trojan horse, where they begin to throw off the entire hormonal system. Xenoestrogens bind to estrogen receptors and can predispose a woman to estrogen dominance, premenopausal symptoms, and even cancer.

Since most xenoestrogens are nonbiodegradable, as a woman gets older they tend to become increasingly concentrated in her fatty tissues. Ever-increasing exposure to xenoestrogens could be one reason we are seeing an increase in breast cancer.

Xenohormones can be found in the following:

- Alcohol
- Fingernail polish
- Fingernail polish remover
- Paints
- Varnishes
- Industrial cleaners
- Degreasers
- Glues
- Dry-cleaning fluids
- Pesticides
- Herbicides
- Plastics
- PCBs (certain toxic chemical compounds)
- Emulsifiers in cosmetics and soaps

These chemicals fool the body into thinking they are estrogen by binding to estrogen receptors, which can then create the symptoms of estrogen dominance.

Chronic constipation can also lead to higher estrogen levels because both xenoestrogens and regular estrogens can be reabsorbed back into the body.

Estrogen as an agricultural additive.

Growth hormones and estrogens are given to animals to fatten them up for market. People eat the meat and this might be a reason for earlier menarche and heavier, taller children in recent decades.

Anyone who has traveled through farm country has probably enjoyed picture-perfect scenes of healthy fat cows and other livestock grazing in the pastures throughout this great country of ours. What does not meet the eye is the fact that most of these animals are much larger and fatter than nature ever intended. Estrogen and other hormones are commonly given to livestock in order to fatten them up. American farmers routinely use hormones, including estrogen, progesterone, and testosterone, so that the cattle will grow faster, larger, and produce more milk and more meat.

In addition, xenohormones are commonly present in the feed. These synthetic hormones become concentrated in the fatty tissues of the animals we eat. This could be why many women are suffering with mood swings and PMS pain and discomfort.

PMS (Premenstrual Syndrome)

As many as 90 percent of premenopausal women suffer some degree of PMS at some point in their lifetime, and about 5 percent of them experience severe PMS. The symptoms can last from two days to as long as two weeks and include headache, mood swings, nausea, acne, bloating, irritability, fatigue, tender breasts, anxiety, depression, low back pain, and more. PMS is caused by the hormonal shift in estrogen/progesterone levels during the menstrual cycle.

Symptoms will resolve near the end of a woman's menstrual period—only to resume within two or three weeks.

SYMPTOMS OF PMS

Weight gain	Low backaches
Breast tenderness	Body aches
Bloating	Nausea
Mood swings	Diarrhea
Irritability	Difficulty sleeping
Acne	Difficulty concentrating, remembering, staying on task
Fatigue	Craving sweet or salty foods
Decreased sex drive	Headaches

Every woman is different in the type of symptoms they experience, but all share the common timing of their symptoms.

Dysmenorrhea (Painful Periods)

Menstrual cramps are common, especially during the first few days of the cycle. Chemicals called prostaglandins are released that stimulate the muscles in the uterus to contract. Over-the-counter pain medications such as ibuprofen block prostaglandins and can be helpful in relieving this pain. It is uncommon to experience pain with the first three to six menstrual cycles, before ovulation is established.

Dysmenorrhea is more common during the early reproductive years and causes significant disruption in life in 15 percent of women.[2] Primary dysmenorrhea is pain without an anatomic cause, while secondary dysmenorrhea results from an abnormality within the uterus. In primary dysmenorrhea there is an excess production of prostaglandins. Symptoms include:

- "Laborlike" pains in the lower abdomen that come and go
- Fatigue
- Low backache
- Headache
- Nausea
- Vomiting
- Diarrhea

Some women use a heating pad on the lower abdomen in an attempt to gain relief from the pain. Nonsteroidal anti-inflammatory drugs (NSAIDs) are often prescribed for symptom relief.

Treatment of PMS Symptoms

PMS treatment is directed toward the symptoms. There is some evidence that a multivitamin with folic acid and calcium supplementation can help. Aerobic exercise, relaxation techniques such as yoga, and dietary changes such as avoiding caffeine, salt, refined sugars, and alcohol are beneficial.

A diet rich in complex carbohydrates and low in simple sugars seems to decrease the irritability of the nervous system. Similarly, decreasing alcohol and caffeine consumption during those two weeks also helps. Exercising several times a week releases endorphins that have a calming effect on the brain. Lessening salt intake can decrease bloating.

Supplements such as calcium, magnesium, and vitamins B_6 and E have been medically proven to aid PMS. In fact, many of the symptoms of PMS are very similar to those seen with calcium deficiency. Some have wondered if a deficiency in calcium explains the development of PMS in some women. Calcium in doses of 1,200 milligrams per day is recommended for those who try this approach. Because calcium is needed to maintain good bone health, it is a helpful supplement regardless of its usefulness in overcoming PMS symptoms.

Magnesium is a mineral that has been shown to calm the nervous system. Obstetricians often administer it intravenously to stop premature labor or to protect women with toxemia from having seizures. Magnesium at 200 milligrams per day has been shown to lessen symptoms of PMS.[3]

Supplements of vitamins B_6 (no more than 100 milligrams per day) and E (400–800 international units) are also helpful, as are herbal remedies including evening primrose, chaste tree berry, and dong quai.[4]

Some women have found that simply understanding the variations of their bodies lessens the impact of PMS. Purposely postponing difficult decisions and angry responses for a few days may be the answer to the confusion and frustration some experience.

LIGHTEN UP

Many women with PMS have depressive symptoms similar to those experienced by people with SAD (seasonal affective disorder). This condition starts most often in the winter or fall. But when a woman with SAD increases her amount of exposure to sunlight, SAD symptoms simply vanish.

Interestingly PMS works similarly for some individuals. The solution is to get out of doors more often. Too many offices have no windows, and workers leave for work in the dark and drive back home in the dark. That leaves noon hours as the most likely time to soak up a little sunshine and get away from the stress of the day.

PMDD (Premenstrual Dysphoric Disorder)

PMDD is a variation of PMS. This is the more severe form of PMS that affects about 5 percent of women.

PMDD requires specific criteria to make the diagnosis, including at least five of the following symptoms beginning in the two weeks prior to menses and ending within four days of the start of the menstrual flow:[5]

- Feeling hopeless or sad
- Feeling tense, anxious, or "on edge"
- Moodiness or frequent crying

- Constant irritability or anger
- Lack of interest in things that are normally enjoyable
- Difficulty concentrating
- Appetite changes, overeating, or cravings
- Trouble sleeping
- Feeling overwhelmed
- Physical symptoms such as swollen breasts, headaches, bloating, and weight gain

PMDD is usually treated with antidepressant medications called selective serotonin reuptake inhibitors (SSRIs). Often treatment begins with birth control pills to smooth the hormonal variations that occur in the second half of the menstrual cycle. These can lessen menstrual cramps and decrease irritability as well. There is even a birth control pill that includes a diuretic (or "water pill") to aid the physical symptoms of bloating and water retention. It is called Yaz and is the only FDA-approved oral contraceptive for the treatment of PMDD. (Special note: This drug appears to have serious side effects.)

> Certain lifestyle changes are recommended to all women who suffer from PMS, such as decreasing caffeine intake and increasing exercise levels.

Most women begin suffering PMS in their twenties and thirties, with symptoms actually worsening in the premenopausal period. PMS fades with menopause. While medical science has not identified the cause of PMS, it is no longer thought to be "only in their heads." Research has speculated that progesterone variations, endorphin changes, or prostaglandin levels interact at a particular time of the month to manifest dozens of signs and symptoms. No two women experience the exact same symptoms, and there is no set treatment that works for everyone.

Natural Supplements Can Help

Data are beginning to accumulate on the value of certain supplements as effective treatments for PMS.

Calcium

For years doctors have observed one interesting association that has not been understood. Women who suffered from PMS when they were younger had a much higher risk of developing osteoporosis as they grew older. As it turns out, calcium is probably the common deficiency in both premenstrual syndrome and osteoporosis. Not surprisingly, then, calcium supplements are an effective treatment for the troubling symptoms of PMS.

The most convincing data on the benefits of supplements for PMS consistently point to calcium supplementation. Women who take 1,000 to 1,200 milligrams of calcium daily have a significant reduction in premenstrual symptoms. To be safe, women (and men as well) should supplement their diets with a total of 1,000 milligrams of calcium in four different forms—the citrate, carbonate, ascorbate and gluconate forms.

Vitamins and minerals

Some studies have also suggested benefits in taking supplements of magnesium at a dose of 400 milligrams daily and vitamin E at a dose of 400–800 international units daily. Vitamin B_6 (75 milligrams per day) has also been widely used for PMS; especially due to its preventive benefits against stroke and heart disease.

Chasteberry

One herbal supplement that can be very useful in alleviating symptoms of premenstrual syndrome is the herb vitex, also known as chasteberry. Decreased PMS symptoms were noted in 70 to 80 percent of the women who used this herbal supplement, which tends to increase the levels of progesterone in the body in a natural way.

MENSTRUAL CYCLE SUPPLEMENTS

- **Quercetin** is a potent antioxidant that reduces the inflammation of endometriosis. It also helps reduce estrogen and cholesterol levels, while boosting circulation and proper digestion.
- **Chasteberry** promotes progesterone production.
- **Bromelain** is a digestive enzyme that reduces pain and inflammation when taken between meals.
- **Essential fatty acids** help to reduce pain due to bloating, breast tenderness, endometriosis, and menstrual cramping. They are also good for skin, hair, and the heart.
- **Vitamin C**. Taking 600–2,000 milligrams daily (divided doses) can help fight heart disease by preventing LDL oxidation.

Not Ovulating Leads to a Progesterone Deficit

Although they may be completely unaware of it, many women have stopped ovulating even while they continue to have regular monthly periods. If a woman doesn't ovulate, her body misses a beat and the hormonal balance is disrupted. It is like trying to play a musical score without a major instrument—the orchestration lacks a significant part.

Without ovulation, the corpus luteum is not formed, so a woman ends up without enough progesterone. Here are some factors that can suspend ovulation:

- Too much stress
- Poor nutrition, sometimes stemming from eating disorders such as anorexia
- Exposure to xenohormones or xenoestrogens, man-made chemicals with hormonal effects
- Inadequate amounts of the necessary vitamins, minerals, and enzymes to convert one hormone to another

Certain medications for psychiatric or neurological conditions also have an impact on ovulation because of their effect on the signals sent by the brain.

Causative factors

Excessive stress is commonly associated with anovulatory cycles in which a woman doesn't ovulate and, thus, doesn't produce enough progesterone. Let's look at what can contribute to not ovulating.

Lack of balance. Too much or too little estrogen, testosterone, cortisol, progesterone or any of the intermediate hormones, such as pregnenolone and DHEA, can disrupt a body's delicate balance.

Too much exercise. Although it's not a problem for most of us, too much physical exercise can be as detrimental as too little. The rigorous physical lifestyles of some female athletes, such as long-distance runners, can cause them to stop ovulating.

Too busy. Excessive mental stress works the same way. In our fast-paced society many women shoulder too many responsibilities, juggling full-time employment with serving as taxi-driver for the kids; full-time cook, laundry, and cleaning lady, Cub Scout mom—and the list goes on and on. There simply aren't enough hours in a day for all of the activities that many attempt to do. Before long, sleep becomes seriously compromised, and hormonal troubles flare up. Over time the rigors of such lifestyles take a real toll upon a woman's mind and body, and one result can be the cessation of ovulation. PMS symptoms could actually be the body's way of signaling, "Take it a little slower!"

Too emotionally wrung out. Emotional stress can also do the same. The death of a loved one, a divorce, dealing with a child with ADD, dealing with children on drugs, anxiety, and depression can cause excessive stress, resulting in anovulatory cycles.

When a woman stops ovulating and her hormones become unbalanced because too little progesterone is being produced, the hormone estrogen becomes dominant.

The progesterone in a woman's body can be converted to cortisol, which is similar to cortisone, and it can also be transformed, directly or indirectly, into other hormones, including testosterone, estrogen, and aldosterone. The higher levels of cortisol that are produced when a person is under a great deal of stress depend on the body having enough progesterone. If a woman has stopped ovulating and her progesterone levels have decreased, then her body may not be able to produce enough cortisol. That's why, over time, low progesterone levels can eventually lead to chronic fatigue and exhaustion. A lack of cortisol will lead to low blood sugar, allergies, immune dysfunction, and arthritis as well. Aldosterone helps the body to maintain the correct balance of minerals. Obviously it is all important to a woman's health to have the proper levels of these steroid hormones.

Other Menstrual Cycle Problems

Dysfunctional uterine bleeding (DUB) is defined as excessively heavy, prolonged, or frequent bleeding that is not caused by a uterine abnormality, but rather by hormonal alterations. Heavy menstrual periods are defined by either the amount of blood lost, known as menorrhagia, or an excessive number of days (more than seven) bleeding (polymenorrhea). A woman has menorrhagia if the blood loss exceeds 80 milliliter, and one way to quantify this is by how frequently she must change a tampon or sanitary pad. More often than every hour while awake is too much bleeding. Passing large clots can also be a sign of heavy bleeding. It is normal to pass clots, as long as they are no larger than a dime.

DUB is a common problem at the "bookends" of a woman's reproductive life—at the beginning and the end. In anovulatory cycles the estrogen levels rise as usual, but since an egg is not released, a corpus luteum is never formed. Therefore, progesterone is not produced. The endometrium continues to proliferate and eventually outgrows its blood supply. This leads to irregular bleeding as part of the lining is sloughed.

Polycystic ovarian syndrome (PCOS) is a medical condition that affects young women at the beginning of their reproductive lives. PCOS causes weight gain after puberty. The cause of PCOS is unknown but is primarily an endocrine (hormone) disorder. In PCOS the ovaries do not ovulate properly, creating cysts that secrete too much testosterone, which leads to increased acne and thickening of facial, chest, and abdominal hair. Male-pattern baldness can also occur over time.

There is also an increase in insulin production, which encourages deposits into the fat cells, leading to rapid increases in weight during the teens and early twenties. At the same time, the hormonal imbalance stops ovulation, resulting in irregular or even absent menstrual periods and later infertility. Women who suffer from PCOS have an increased lifetime risk of diabetes as they become insensitive to insulin. High cholesterol levels lead to an increased risk of heart disease. PCOS is a serious condition, affecting nearly 10 percent of all women.[6]

Because the hallmark traits of this disease are weight gain, acne, facial hair, and irregular menstrual cycles, women with PCOS suffer from poor self-esteem and body image. They feel they have no control over their bodies and watch themselves gain weight while typically eating far less than their peers. The cosmetic changes these teens and young adults experience will be with them for life.

PCOS can be treated with birth control pills to put the ovaries at "rest" and stop the imbalance that is occurring. This will regulate the menstrual cycle and stop further unwanted hair growth. A brand that is specifically designed for PCOS is called Yasmin. It has a mild diuretic that daily flushes out the water retention and bloating commonly experienced by patients during their menstrual cycles. The progesterone component is unique in that it does not digest itself into any testosterone-like by-products, which helps with the acne and facial hair complaints. Women who take Yasmin should be aware, however, of possible unwanted side effects.

The cosmetic changes that have already occurred that involve facial and body hair are more difficult to eliminate. Some dermatologists prescribe medication to stop hair growth. These take many months to work as each hair follicle has a long lifespan. For those wanting faster results, laser hair removal has become a popular alternative, but it is expensive for some and requires multiple treatments.

PCOS is a common reason women do not ovulate. There is speculation that local insulin levels may be too high and that they suppress ovulation. Body fat stores estrogen and sends false messages to the brain that estrogen levels are sufficient, altering the signals sent by the brain to the ovaries to spur ovulation. Thyroid disease can send similar false signals from the brain, which disrupt ovulation.

Making It All Work

Perhaps the most common forms of emotional disorders treated by OB/GYN specialists that relate to hormonal imbalances in women are PMS, PMDD, depression, and generalized anxiety disorder (GAD). OB/GYN doctors have not specialized in the field of psychology or mental health, but they do work with these specialists to help patients regain their lives.

All menstrual disorders respond to the right combination of approaches, although often a period of trial and error precedes success. Of course a woman's body is always changing as well, so new approaches may be required as time goes on.

Chapter 5

PREMENOPAUSE, MENOPAUSE, POSTMENOPAUSE

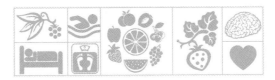

I**N THE INTRODUCTION** we compared the seasons of a woman's life to the seasons of the year. These seasons of a woman's life, like the seasons of the year, revolve around her reproductive capabilities. Spring is the coming-of-age season, when everything wakes up—beautifully; a woman's femininity awakens in the tender bloom of her youth. Summer is the fruitful time, when babies are born and families are nurtured. Autumn is harvest time, a time of joyful preparation for the bedding-down and resting of winter, a season when the harvest of all the good things a woman has planted into those around her comes back to her.

Just as "summer," when a woman's hormone production is in full swing, precedes the autumn, so premenopause (often known as perimenopause) blends into the transitional time known as menopause. The experience of menopause varies from one woman to another, depending on a multiplicity of interacting factors. But—unless it is induced by surgery—it certainly does not occur overnight. Following a woman's final menstrual period, which can only be determined in retrospect after months of cessation in her up-to-then monthly cycle we say she is "postmenopausal." Women who have not had a menstrual cycle for a year are considered postmenopausal.

Premenopause

Premenopause (or perimenopause) begins after the age of forty and continues until sometime in the fifties, when a woman's menstrual period becomes a thing of the past. Premenopause signals the beginning of menopause. Starting at about forty, a thorough OB/GYN will perform baseline tests such as cholesterol, mammography, and colonoscopy, and screenings for osteoporosis, heart disease, and diabetes.

During this stage of life, many women experience a decrease or even cessation in their progesterone production because of irregular ovarian cycling and ovarian aging. At the same time, estrogen levels may be comparatively high, causing a troubling state of continual imbalance that is now recognized as "estrogen dominance," which results in a plethora of symptoms, including the following:

- Fatigue
- Breast tenderness
- Foggy thinking
- Irritability
- Headaches
- Insomnia
- Allergy symptoms (including asthma)
- Fat gain—especially around the middle

- Mood swings
- Memory loss, difficulty concentrating
- Water retention
- Bone loss
- Slowed metabolism
- Decreased sex drive
- Anxiety, depression

One of the first symptoms will be irregular periods. A woman may have two or three normal periods, and then skip one or two, or a period may come at an unexpected time. Then she may notice stranger symptoms: hot flashes and night sweats are among the most common. She may not be aware of more subtle changes that are taking place, such as vascular changes in the eye that begin to cause a fuzziness in her vision. Some women experience a crawling sensation on their skin, as though an insect were crawling on their arm, but when they look, there is nothing there. Urinary tract infections increase as vaginal dryness increases. And one especially troubling symptom that is caused by a decrease in the female hormones is an increasing loss of scalp hair, along with the development of hair in other parts of their body.

Premenopause, the time of transition from normal menstrual cycles to the complete absence of cycles, generally lasts for four to seven years. This is often the time period women refer to when they complain of "going through menopause." After the early phase, usually in the forties, where menstrual cycles begin to become irregular, the later phase begins (in the late forties or early fifties), signified by missed cycles and menopausal symptoms. The quality of the eggs not "chosen" earlier in life is poorer and results in lower estrogen levels. This in turns prevents consistent ovulation of the egg and causes weak progesterone levels. The lower progesterone levels lead to irregular or missed menstrual cycles.

It is very rare to abruptly stop having periods and never have them again. For most women the transition from fertility to menopause is an inconsistent and unpredictable one. Cycles can be closer together or farther apart. They can be shorter than usual or longer and heavier. It is most important to consult your doctor if your periods become extremely heavy, last longer than seven days, occur closer than twenty-one days apart, or if there is bleeding after intercourse. Sometimes bleeding can occur between periods and may need evaluation as well. (Any bleeding in the postmenopausal period, after twelve months or more of no menses, requires investigation for the possibility of uterine or cervical cancer.)

Some of the tools that can be used to evaluate abnormal bleeding are ultrasonography or sonohysterography to look for polyps or fibroids. Endometrial biopsy can sample the lining of the uterus to exclude precancerous or cancerous changes. Hysteroscopy is a surgical tool to look directly into the uterus for abnormalities. Other conditions can cause irregular menstrual bleeding or missed periods, such as thyroid disease, that may need evaluation.

Natural Progesterone

Hormonal imbalance has far-reaching effects on many tissues in the body, including the heart, brain, blood vessels, bones, uterus, and breasts. If the levels of estrogen and progesterone can be brought back into balance, the pathway of premenopause will be smoother. It is an undeniable blessing for a woman to feel wonderful again—vital, alert, optimistic, sociable, and nurturing toward themselves and others.

Natural (nature-identical or bioidentical) progesterone can balance the ratio of estrogen and progesterone in a woman's body, thereby alleviating all of the symptoms of estrogen dominance. In addition it helps to build bone and relieve anxiety. It may also protect against breast cancer.[1] Typically natural progesterone is compounded as a cream.

> **Q:** Do nature-identical hormones put me at the same risk as traditional pharmaceutical versions?
>
> **A:** Quite honestly this question cannot be answered. Other than the greater lipid-protective benefits, ability to reduce hot flashes, and its lower side-effect profile, micronized (nature-identical) progesterone is about the only "natural" hormone with some support in the scientific literature. Most estrogen products, whether from a large pharmaceutical house or a compounding pharmacy, are soy-based, and many prefer the weakest form of estrogen, estriol. As an alternative to seeking a "new" estrogen, others use lifestyle changes, therapeutic nutrition, and botanicals.

The following guidelines for using progesterone cream are based upon a 2-ounce container containing 960 milligrams total. Areas of application include chest, inner arms, neck, face, palms, and even the soles of the feet if they are not calloused. Women should rotate through the places they apply the cream, changing them every day, applying it in the morning and again at bedtime.[2] Women who still have their ovaries and uterus should apply the cream as follows:

- After ovulation (days 14–18 after onset of last period): a small amount of cream, no more than ¼ teaspoon, once daily.

- Days 18–23: use ¼ teaspoon twice daily, gradually increasing to ½ teaspoon twice daily.

- Day 23 to start of period: use ½ teaspoon twice daily.

Women without ovaries due to hysterectomy should apply progesterone cream as follows:

- ¼–½ teaspoon of progesterone cream twice daily for twenty-five days of the calendar month, going five to seven days without it.

- Women with endometriosis should use the progesterone cream on days 8–26 of their cycles.

- Women who have ovaries but no uterus should use ¼–½ teaspoon twice a day for three weeks out of the month.

- Premenopausal women who are menstruating but not ovulating should use ¼–½ teaspoon daily, beginning use on day 10–12 of their cycles and continuing until their expected period, when they stop, until day 10–12 again.

Some women notice results right away. Others may see positive changes in one to three months. A woman who notices unpleasant symptoms prior to ovulation (for example, migraines or moodiness) may want to begin using the cream earlier, until her period begins. Progesterone is not usually used during menstruation, but women who experience cramps or other symptoms during menstruation may use the cream until the symptoms are alleviated.

Menopause

You're fifty-plus. You're gaining weight, your periods have stopped, you have been diagnosed with uterine fibroids, your breasts are sore and lumpy, your skin has changed and lacks that velvety texture, your sex drive has decreased, you're irritable, you're anxious, and you're maybe even depressed. You would do anything for a good night's sleep. It is the time to fasten your seatbelt, because the roller-coaster ride is about to begin: you have reached menopause!

Today menopausal women find themselves at a crossroads. Should they take estrogen for the sometimes-debilitating pains of menopause—and risk hormone-related cancer later on—or do they suffer in silence as their bodies ache and rapidly age? Should they live in a hormone-deficient state and subject themselves to the possibility of acquiring the degenerative diseases that attack a body that lacks proper balance?

Menopause is a challenging time in a woman's life physically, emotionally, sexually, and spiritually.

> The most prominent hormonal change of menopause is a dramatic re-duction in circulating estradiol levels. The symptom most clearly linked to menopause is hot flashes. The most prominent complaint associated with menopause is joint aches and pain.[3]

In the Western world the average age of menopause is fifty-one, with the ages from forty to fifty-eight encompassing the natural statistical curve. Menopause before age forty is considered "premature," whether it happened spontaneously (i.e., naturally) or through surgery, chemotherapy, or radiation. Every woman who lives long enough will proceed through this phase of life called menopause.

Menopause is defined as the period of time when the available eggs in the ovary have dwindled and the estrogen levels have dropped dramatically. Menopause has fully arrived when a year has passed since a woman's last period and certain blood levels signify the end of ovarian function. Medically it is a set moment in time. But for most women the process leading up to it can last several years. All of life after menopause is termed "postmenopausal."

With the completion of menopause comes amenorrhea or loss of menstruation. The cessation of menstrual periods is a blessing for most, but it also signals the end of fertility. While it is rare to find a woman who still wants to have a child in her fifties, the very fact that she can never have one again can bring a time of mourning. Even women who have had a tubal ligation years earlier find that they become sad when the last egg is gone. Their hormonal and physiological processes have been geared toward fertility and childbearing. Now they must face the realization that new life will no longer come from their wombs. For some this calls for a radical reshaping of their self-image. For others this simply means that they are getting "old."

On the positive side the lack of menstruation frees a woman to be sexually active whenever she wants. She will no longer be a victim of some ill-timed blood flow or painful menstrual cramps. Freedom! Birth control is not an issue or a burden. Sex can be for fun instead of carrying the fear of unwanted pregnancy. The ovaries continue to produce a small amount of weak estrogen, and the production of testosterone continues. With the balance of hormone shifted to the male side, some women even have an increase in libido after menopause is completed.

Hot flashes

As women enter menopause, there will be about 15 percent who experience no symptoms at all except a loss of menstruation. They will not complain of hot flashes or mood swings or anything their fellow sisters in menopause are going through. In fact, they may have a difficult time understanding what the other 85 percent are experiencing. But the majority of women will have varying degrees of difficulty as they transition through this phase of life. How much it bothers them will determine what remedies they seek.

TIPS FOR DEALING WITH HOT FLASHES

- When a hot flash starts, go somewhere cool or touch something cold.
- Sleeping in a cool room or with a fan on may keep hot flashes from waking you up during the night.
- Dress in layers that you can take off if you get warm.
- Use sheets and clothing that let your skin "breathe."
- Try having a cold drink of water or juice at the beginning of a hot flash.

At the beginning of menopause, nightly hot flashes are the most bothersome, making women wake up in the middle of the night, often covered in sweat, only to become cold again. This repeated interruption in sleep patterns causes fatigue and poor concentration during the day.

As menopause progresses, the hot flashes begin to intrude upon the daytime hours. They can be socially embarrassing, with facial flushing, sweating, and feeling hot when no one else in the room does. The core body temperature does not actually increase, but the skin temperature can raise four to seven degrees in a matter of seconds, only to plummet again a few moments later.

No one knows what causes hot flashes, but some speculate that hot flashes come from an area in the brain called the hypothalamus, which is the temperature regulation center. Signals may be sent from this center that dilate blood vessels on the skin in an attempt to cool the body, leading to the "flushed" sensation that often begins in the torso and spreads upward. This can occur several times an hour or only a few times a day. It generally stops occurring a few years postmenopausal, but some women continue to experience hot flashes into their seventies.

THE DARK SIDE OF SOY

Soy in its most natural form (organic, not genetically modified) is a complete protein that can stand on its own. This is because, despite being considered a legume or bean, it contains all the essential amino acids to make it a complete protein. Fermented soy such as tofu, miso soup, tempeh, and natto are easily digested and assimilated. Soy has been proven to lower cholesterol, diminish the risk of myocardial infarction (MI) and heart disease, decrease hot flashes in menopausal women, and may prevent both memory loss and breast cancer.

Unfortunately, there is a potential dark side of soy, as recent and somewhat controversial research indicates. Many scientists now believe that overconsuming soy may do more harm than good. High consumption of isoflavones, which are the estrogen-like plant chemicals contained in soy, may stimulate the production of breast cancer cells. It may also increase the chances of developing serious reproductive, thyroid, and liver problems.[5]

Besides this, most soy products are processed and have a low biological value compared to other proteins—meaning the body doesn't use them very efficiently. This includes two of the most commonly consumed soy products, soy milk and soy protein. These products can interfere with thyroid functioning and lower the metabolic rate, making it more difficult to lose weight. In general, there are many adults and children on soy milk or soy protein powder, and it may be doing them more harm than good, especially if they are trying to lose weight.

To give you a better picture, 90 percent of all soy sold in the United States is genetically modified (GM). Soy is also one of the top seven allergens. Studies have shown that the healthy benefits Asian people experience by consuming soy is because they consume natural or fermented soy, not the highly processed versions.

If you enjoy soy, it is recommended that you try cutting back or eliminating soy products altogether. Know this: the final word on soy is not yet in. Even the soy skeptics say the bottom line is to opt for natural forms of soy rather than chemically altered or genetically modified (GM). Because it remains a somewhat controversial protein, it is advised to proceed with caution. Do not eat or drink soy products every day; if you must consume soy, do it only a couple times a week.

Certain natural, herbal preparations can help with hot flashes, such as soy, red clover, and black cohosh. Soy is a main dietary ingredient in the Orient, and many of those cultures lack a word for "hot flashes." Because the typical American diet is not rich in soy, most women must boost their soy intake with supplements. This dietary supplement is safe but fairly weak in its ability to reduce hot flashes.

Soy has two primary isoflavones, genistein being the most prominent, and red clover has four, so when these two are taken in combination with each other, the results are powerful. While soy mimics the diet of most Asian cultures, red clover contains many of the properties of the legumes found in Mediterranean countries, such as beans and chickpeas. In both of these cultures menopausal symptoms are rare.

Soy is what is called a "selective estrogen receptor modulator," which simply means that it blocks the receptor sites that would generally bind with the prescription estrogen and cause either breast or uterine cancer. Studies show that women who are taking higher doses of soy isoflavones demonstrate a 54 percent decrease in uterine cancer. The same is true of heart disease.[4]

The FDA allows soy to make a "heart protective claim," based on the many studies that show its role in decreasing the LDL (bad) cholesterol and increasing the HDL (good) cholesterol levels. Also the genistein present in both soy and red clover inhibits the breakdown of bone in the body and stimulates the formation of new bone. Fifty milligrams daily of the soy isoflavones and 500 milligrams daily of red clover leaf extract will bring the greatest benefit.

Black cohosh was used for centuries by American Indian women to relieve menopausal symptoms and is widely used in Europe, where it has been approved by their regulatory board for the use in treating vasomotor symptoms (hot flashes and night sweats). In the United States the most popular brand is made by a large pharmaceutical company under the name Remifemin. Doses of 40–80 milligrams per day have been shown to be effective in reducing hot flashes for many women.[6] It seems that women who have been the most satisfied with herbal remedies have been those with milder vasomotor symptoms. There do not appear to be any long-term side effects to black cohosh except very rare cases of liver disease.

Black cohosh is a phytoestrogen (estrogen derived from a plant) that comes from a buttercup plant. The chemicals within the black cohosh, such as soy and red clover, bind to the estrogen receptor sites. Black cohosh also seems to alleviate headaches, heart palpitations, depression and anxiety, and vaginal dryness and atrophy, thus preventing urinary tract infections. It also helps alleviate dizziness, high blood pressure, and high blood sugar.[7]

ESSENTIAL NUTRIENTS TO EASE THE DISCOMFORTS OF MENOPAUSE		
Natural Substance	Effect	Daily Dosage
Red clover leaf extract	Herb rich in isoflavones that helps balance hormones, promote healthy bones, and support cardiovascular function	500 milligrams
Dong quai root extract	Herb traditionally used to support hormonal balance in women	300 milligrams
Siberian ginseng root extract	Member of the ginseng family traditionally used in both China and Russia to help increase resistance to stress, fatigue, and illness	200 milligrams
Black cohosh root extract	Herb rich in phytosterols that has been used traditionally to help support hormonal balance	80 milligrams
Soy isoflavones	Natural compounds from soy that help regulate hormone balance and support skeletal and cardiovascular health	50 milligrams
Bromelain	Enzyme derived from pineapple that helps with the digestion and absorption of nutrients	45 milligrams
Boron	Mineral that helps strengthen bones and cartilage	3 milligrams

Some serotonin agents previously used for depression have been found to improve hot flashes and are often prescribed to women who have had breast cancer and cannot take estrogen. In one study the drug Paxil produced a drop in hot flashes by 67 percent.[8]

Other symptoms of menopause

Decreasing estrogen levels have been linked to increasing irritability, depression, sleep deprivation, and loss of memory. No definitive studies have established estrogen loss as the cause, although women who have surgically lost their ovaries seem to experience these symptoms at a greater level than those who enter menopause gradually. The presence of hot flashes and night sweats can disrupt the normal sleep patterns. Poor sleep in turn leads to irritability, depression, and poor concentration.

Sleep aids range from herbal (valerian root), to antihistamine (Simply Sleep, Unisom, Tylenol PM), to prescription (Ambien, Lunesta, Rozerem). The latter can be troublesome in long-term use and require the supervision of a physician.

The lack of estrogen to the vagina leads to thinning of the vaginal lining and dryness. This in turn causes painful intercourse. Estrogen loss changes vaginal pH and its microorganisms, making it more difficult to defend against yeast or bacterial infections. The ligaments that hold the female organs in place can weaken, letting the bladder, uterus, or rectum prolapse into the vagina, bringing discomfort with standing or during intercourse. Bladder control can be partially lost, leading to wetness or urinary tract infections. An overactive bladder, which makes women always feel the need to urinate, may develop. While these changes may not be specifically tied to hormone loss, they are frequent menopausal complaints.

Hormone supplements—yes or no?

The main question that comes with menopause is whether or not to take hormone supplements. Of all the remedies known to mankind, nothing relieves hot flashes and night sweats like estrogen. It is the hormone that the body is crying out for, and every other remedy is a pale substitute. Estrogen used to be prescribed to almost every menopausal woman in the United States at some point in her life. It was thought for decades that estrogen would prevent heart disease, strokes, osteoporosis, and certain cancers, while improving the quality of life for those suffering from hot flashes and mood swings.

This prescribing pattern came to an abrupt end in 2002. That was when the Women's Health Initiative (WHI), a large national study of thousands of women, stopped its study of hormone replacement therapy (HRT) early because it was finding that the women who were taking hormones were doing worse than the women who were taking placebo (or fake) pills. (See chapter 3 for more information.) The body of evidence had shown that HRT, specifically estrogen, was beneficial in raising "good" cholesterol and lowering "bad" cholesterol; it was assumed that this would indicate an improvement for the heart. Therefore, HRT was recommended as a way to prevent heart attacks and strokes. Since most women did not suffer cardiac events until after menopause, it was thought that female hormones protected women and that replacing them could continue this "fountain of youth."

Studies were designed to test these theories. When instead they revealed unknown dangers of HRT, the studies were suspended and doctors immediately stopped advocating hormones as a preventative treatment for heart disease and other diseases. The sale of Premarin, which had been the most prescribed drug in the United States, dropped precipitously overnight. It was once hoped that estrogen could prevent the development of dementia or Alzheimer's disease. But the WHI also showed that estrogen used over many years can actually increase the risk of dementia, probably through a series of undiagnosed strokes.

Although reanalysis of the data and subsequent studies have revealed certain disease-related benefits of HRT, the only proven benefits of both estrogen and progesterone include relief of hot flashes, night sweats, vaginal dryness, and pain with intercourse. In fact, no other drugs come close to providing the kind of relief that HRT and ERT can provide for these symptoms. Hormone replacement therapy also helps prevent osteoporosis in the hip and spine.

From an FDA standpoint, estrogen and progesterone are approved for short-term use (ideally, less than five years) in the treatment of moderate to severe hot flashes, night sweats, and osteoporosis prevention. Women with a uterus should have progesterone added to their estrogen to prevent uterine cancer. Women who do not have a uterus should be on estrogen alone, as the addition of progesterone offers no benefits and the potential for more complications.

> Typical clinical changes of menopause include menstrual irregularities four years before, hormonal changes eight years before, and a decline in fertility up to ten years before menses cease.[9]

The Estrogen-Osteoporosis Connection

Millions of women suffer from osteoporosis and have sustained vertebral fractures that cause hunched spines, or hip fractures that have left them bound to a walker or wheelchair. A visit to any nursing home in America will reveal hallways lined with old women who are immobile and dependent on others even to take them to the bathroom. Much of this could have been prevented by better bone health as they aged.

Estrogen is a powerful preventative of spine and hip fractures. For the longest time it was the only preventative we had that could take calcium and bind it back into the bones. But new drugs have been developed that not only prevent osteoporosis but also can reverse some of the bone loss that has already taken place. Some of these agents even appear to prevent breast cancer and may decrease the risk of heart disease. These new "designer" drugs called SERMs are targeting the areas that need help without the side effects of HRT. With the advent of such therapy, the need for HRT is greatly diminishing.

But the new drugs also cause hot flashes, unwelcome news for menopausal women for whom hot flashes may already be the worst part of menopause. For a woman who has had a sudden loss of estrogen through hysterectomy, hot flashes will be even more severe.

For women with severe hot flashes or mood swings, there is nothing like estrogen to make them feel "normal" again. If the current data holds true, there is no harm in taking HRT for a few years to aid in the transition of menopause until the hot flashes subside. This is, of course, provided you have not had breast cancer or heart disease before. Only your doctor can review your individual history and advise you on your options.

Bioidentical Hormones for Menopause?

Because much of the research cited earlier focused on drugs such as Premarin that were manufactured from animal sources, as well as synthetics, some believe that plant-based drugs (phytoestrogens) might be more "natural" and thus free of the health concerns such as those raised by the shortened WHI study. Tailoring the dose of drug to the individual patient has also been a strong desire as many women find themselves unsatisfied with traditional dosing regimens for prescription hormones and want the ability to have the compounds adjusted to fit their specific needs. In response, compounding pharmacists combine several hormones into a gel, tablet, or suppository form. These hormones include estrogen, progesterone, testosterone, and DHEA.[10]

To determine the correct combination and dosage for each woman, a saliva test is done to ascertain the woman's current hormone concentrations. While this seems logical and scientific, there are potential problems that should be understood. First, the "normal" range for salivary hormone concentrations is broad, and all practitioners are adjusting doses not based on final levels achieved but on subjective symptom relief. Second, the salivary samples are often shipped to reference labs with no guarantee that the hormone concentrations remain stable during shipping. Unlike blood, saliva is not a stable fluid.

Finally, these compounded drugs have never been tested for serious long-term side effects. Because they are compounded by the pharmacist, the FDA does not require the same warning labels as it does for products made by pharmaceutical companies. This is an oversight, not an endorsement of the safety of the product. Because each "batch" is individualized, the FDA has no way of knowing what a patient is receiving. The government continues to caution that until large studies are done on every potential hormone product (which will never happen), results from the Women's Health Initiative study apply to all HRT preparations.[11]

Estrogen Guidelines

There is nothing quite like estrogen to restore the feelings of well-being and prevent vasomotor symptoms. It is the standard by which every other treatment is compared. If a woman is at low risk (does not have a history of breast or uterine cancer, heart disease, stroke, blood clots, or diabetes) then a short course of estrogen for moderate to severe symptoms is safe and beneficial. If she has a uterus, progesterone must be added to protect against uterine cancer.

Nothing can take the place of a face-to-face consultation with your gynecologist, but here are some general guidelines. First, take the lowest dose for the shortest time needed. Try to finish using estrogen within five years if you can. Some women cannot wean off, and that is understandable. But the majority can be gently weaned down in dose and get off hormones within five years.

The most popular hormone replacements before 2002 were Premarin and Prempro. Prempro is for women with a uterus, and Premarin is for those without one. These are still very good products, but because of the WHI, they have fallen out of favor somewhat. Patients who are doing very well with them should not automatically switch to something else.

While there is no evidence to prove this, some feel that a plant-derived estrogen and progesterone regimen might avoid some of the issues that came from the animal-based hormones of the WHI study. Plant-based hormones are on every insurance formulary in America and are less expensive than paying for the compounding products out of pocket. They come in a variety of forms, including oral pills, creams, patches, vaginal rings, and injectables.

Examples of oral estrogen products are estradiol (generic), estriol (generic), Enjuvia (a brand substitution that is close to Premarin but made from plants), Gynodiol (brand-name estradiol), and Femtrace (brand-name estradiol). For those who need the addition of progesterone to the estrogen tablets, there is Activella, Femhrt, and Angeliq. These are really lower doses of birth control pills that have been on the market for many years. It is thought that since there have been no cardiac or breast issues with low-dose birth control pills, using even lower doses for menopause might be safer. Again this is an unproven theory that may have more to do with the age of the woman taking the products than the product itself.

Some women do not want to take an oral medication or may feel that they are not getting good intestinal absorption from the pills. They may desire a more direct route such as a skin cream in the hopes of maximizing symptom relief. Medically, absorbing the drugs directly into the bloodstream may decrease the risk of blood clots, and the liver is bypassed.

Examples of estrogen creams are Premarin, EstroGel, and Estrasorb. Premarin is usually inserted vaginally, while the last two are spread on the arms or legs like a body lotion. A vaginal ring that is available is called Femring. Patches include Climara and Vivelle. For those who need progesterone added to the estrogen, patches include Climara Pro and CombiPatch.

Some women only need relief of vaginal dryness or painful intercourse and do not want estrogen circulating throughout the bloodstream. Local estrogen can be applied that will not enter the bloodstream and can be safely used even with health conditions that would otherwise prevent estrogen use. These include Premarin cream, Vagifem (a vaginal tablet), and Estring (a vaginal ring). Your gynecologist can help you decide which of the available products may be right for you, at what dose, and for how long.

Smooth Sailing

The menopausal-postmenopausal season is a long one, and women need to learn as much as possible about how they can sail through it as smoothly as possible. By 2015 more than half of American women will be menopausal or postmenopausal. Are you one of them yet?

God's desire for you as you pass through the natural life transition of premenopause, menopause, and postmenopause is to be healthy and renewed, so that you can echo the psalmist who declared, "He fills my life with good things. My youth is renewed like the eagle's!" (Ps. 103:5, NLT).

Chapter 6

MOOD SWINGS—STRESS, ANGER, DEPRESSION, AND ANXIETY

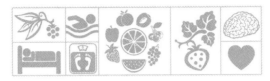

GOD PROMISES HIS people rest and peace—and that includes the women whose hormones may be causing mood swings and unsettling emotional instability. The prophet Isaiah wrote, "You will keep him in perfect peace, whose mind is stayed on You, because he trusts in You" (Isa. 26:3). David, who was a shepherd boy before he became king of Israel, wrote these familiar words:

> The LORD is my shepherd; I have all that I need. He lets me rest in green meadows; he leads me beside peaceful streams. He renews my strength. He guides me along right paths, bringing honor to his name.
> —PSALM 23:1–3, NLT

So in spite of the ups and downs of a woman's life, she can learn how to walk in God's rest, and it is vitally important to do so, spiritually, mentally, and physically. This is more than getting enough sleep, although that is very important. Emotions can be volatile when a woman is exhausted, but getting a good night's rest can be elusive. Simply meditating on the Word of God before bedtime and keeping worship songs flowing throughout the day can begin to help the body dial down and relax. Getting a good night's sleep, along with resting by honoring the Sabbath, are keys to restoring and maintaining a woman's mental, emotional, and physical health.

MELATONIN

Melatonin is an antioxidant hormone. Studies have shown that a nightly melatonin supplement boosts the performance during sleep of immune systems compromised by age, drugs, or stress. It helps to keep us in rhythm with the day and the seasons and reduces sleep disorders.

Stress and Anxiety

A certain amount of stress is normal and necessary in everyone's life. Without the stress of the alarm clock every morning, many of us would fail to get up in time to meet the daily responsibilities. Some women respond better to some stress in their lives than no stress at all. But nearly every woman today has more stressors in her life than is healthy. It is important to take action and determine now to bring more balance into one's life by eliminating some of the mental and physical depletion of stressful days, week after week.

> ### JUST SAY NO
>
> Remember back when you were two years old and how powerful you felt when you said no? Regardless of how old you are now, go ahead and act like a two-year-old and just say no. If you have the "disease to please"—attempting to please everyone—you must learn how to acknowledge your limitations and your need for peace. Saying no to over commitment means saying yes to peace and calm.

When stress is ignored, it can escalate to *distress*. A woman who is distressed is headed for burnout and total exhaustion. Stress is the body's signal that something needs attention. It has been said, "If you do not take the time to be well, you will definitely take the time to be sick." Stress, when not addressed, makes women vulnerable to emotional and physical illness, such as anxiety, illness, heart attacks, and depression. Every woman is different, so the solutions vary accordingly.

A "stressor" is any demand, good or bad, that is made upon a person's body or mind. Stressors can be caused by external pressures, such as a bad work environment, or internal pressures, such as feelings of competitiveness, insecurity, or too much self-sacrifice for the sake of family or others. The place to begin is identifying the specific causes of stress, sometimes by observing the effects it is having on the body, mind, and spirit. Some stressful situations are unchangeable. A woman must stop expending so much of her precious emotional energy on those unalterable situations so that she can begin to focus on areas for which she can find solutions.

Undoing the damage of too much external or internal stress is not like getting over the flu. The process takes a while, and it involves some of the most benign of interventions. While the option exists to change jobs or trim a few things off the weekly schedule by reprioritizing, most women can count on always facing more stress. There will always be family members who expect too much, children who misbehave, and the unrelenting pace of modern life. Without being able to eliminate all stress, we must resist it where we can and learn to live with it in ways that don't hurt us.

STRESS OVERLOAD?

Check each symptom you are experiencing:

❑ Anger   ❑ High blood pressure
❑ Anxiety   ❑ Inability to concentrate
❑ Burnout   ❑ Irritability
❑ Decreased sexual interest ❑ Lack of appetite
❑ Depression   ❑ Muscle tension
❑ Headaches   ❑ Sleeplessness
❑ Indigestion

The benefits of stress-releasing efforts such as therapeutic nutrition, exercise, and social support are overlapping. The stress response is intended to supply energy to respond to a crisis, but working that energy off by walking or going to the gym makes de-stressing easier—except for someone who is at the burnout stage, when less exercise is called for. Regular exercise will go a long way toward helping the body to reclaim its proper hormonal balance. A vital mechanism of exercise that reduces stress is the production and release of natural opiates known as endorphins.

Keep your sense of humor. Laughter releases tension.
Look for what's funny in everyday life.

Other simple interventions that work against stress include, as already mentioned, getting enough rest and relaxation. Relaxation techniques, be they physical or mental, are valuable interventions that reduce the harmful effects of stress. Yoga is effective because of its ability to center and calm, as well as its encouragement to focus on breathing. Just breathing deeply can quell a racing heart and quell stress. There are no side effects or financial costs for this very powerful intervention that can be done anywhere. It is impossible to be anxious at the same time you are breathing deeply, slowly, and regularly.

The restorative actions of prayer and meditation are also well researched. Meditation counteracts the fight-or-flight response at a hormonal level, slows the metabolism of red blood cells, and suppresses the production of cytokines—proteins that generate pro-inflammatory responses in the body. The focus on breathing that is recommended during meditation keeps negative, distracting thoughts away. Massage and aromatherapy are additional calming techniques that help relieve stress.

FOUR LEVELS OF STRESS

Level I

- Losing interest in enjoyable activities
- Sagging of the corners of the eyes
- Creasing of the forehead
- Becoming short-tempered
- Bored, nervous

Level II

- All of level I, plus:
- Tiredness, anger, insomnia, paranoia, sadness

Level III

- All of levels I and II, plus:
- Chronic head and neck aches
- High blood pressure
- Upset stomach
- Looking older

Level IV

- All of levels I, II, and III, plus:
- Skin disorders
- Kidney malfunction
- Frequent infections
- Asthma
- Heart disease
- Mental or emotional breakdown

Studies confirm that people with an active and satisfying social network handle life's ups and down better, especially when they can laugh together. Organizing life so there is time for play and leisure activities is restorative. At the same time, too much of a social life is not a good thing; women must learn to say "no" and to set limits.

Stress-Busting Ideas

At the end of a particularly stressful day, take a soothing aromatherapy bath by candle-light. Fill the tub with steamy hot water and fragrant aromatherapy oil such as lavender. Play some soft, instrumental music and relax. Aromatherapy, or the fragrant use of essential oils, is the way many women prefer to handle the pain, anxiety, and depression that comes with PMS. Smell has a powerful influence on the body and mind, possibly because the olfactory nerve is in direct contact with the emotional center of the brain.

AROMATHERAPY BASICS

- Choose aromatic essential oils (found at health food stores)
- Add 5–10 drops of essential oils to hot water while filling your bath.
- Do not combine essential oils with other bath oils or soap.
- Make sure to soak in the tub for at least 20 minutes to get the aromatic benefits.

Essential oils that are especially beneficial in relieving stressful PMS symptoms:

- **Lavender.** At first this oil may pep you up a little. But as you soak for a few minutes, you'll find that it calms you. It relieves nervous tension, depression, and insomnia.
- **Geranium.** Combine a couple of drops of this with lavender. It has a calming effect.
- **Rosemary.** This one helps circulation. Use it alone or with lavender to relieve depression.

A hot cup of herbal tea can be just what the doctor ordered to calm nerves at stressful moments (using one or two teaspoons of the dry herb for each 8-ounce cup of hot, but not boiling, water, covered and steeped for ten to fifteen minutes). The following teas have a proven track record as stress-busters, especially for women who are under the hormonal stresses of PMS or premenopause:

- Chasteberry tea
- Skullcap tea

- Dong quai tea (known in Chinese lore as the female tonic)
- Specially prepared PMS teas (found at health food and grocery stores)

Some people believe that a woman's level of stress is hormonally linked to her exposure to xenoestrogens. To reduce xenoestrogen exposure, stop using pesticides around your home, as well as all solvents, including alcohol and mineral spirits. Watch out for fingernail polish, industrial cleaners and degreasers, paints, and some air fresheners. For cleaners, choose natural products instead of petrochemical products. Also be careful about drinking hot beverages or eating hot soups from certain types of plastic cups or bowls, and avoid microwaving your food in plastic containers, which is thought to release xenoestrogens.

"I'm stressing and PMS-ing"

High stress raises levels of the hormones cortisol and adrenaline, which lead to decreased levels of progesterone and PMS symptoms. It will also raise the levels of aldosterone, which regulates the minerals in the cells. Too much stress causes the adrenal glands to secrete excessive amounts of aldosterone, which may raise your blood pressure by triggering the kidneys to retain sodium and to excrete potassium and magnesium. This may also lead to water retention, bloating in the abdomen and edema (or swelling) in the lower extremities.

Thus many of the symptoms of PMS are caused by elevated levels of the hormones cortisol, adrenaline, and aldosterone, all of which are triggered by too much stress. Stress also raises the levels of another hormone called prolactin. Prolactin stimulates the breasts to make milk, but it also lowers the production of progesterone.

Calcium helps to alleviate symptoms of premenstrual syndrome by aiding the body in balancing proper hormone levels.

Learning to control or lower the overall stress level is critically important for managing the symptoms of PMS, because a woman can thereby lower the levels of the hormones cortisol, adrenaline, aldosterone, and prolactin. In order to balance hormones you must get a handle on your stress.

Progesterone can help with mood swings. By balancing cortisol levels, progesterone can improve energy level, immune function, allergy resistance, and mental concentration.

Stress junkies

Some people cultivate stress. They create a "crisis of the moment" to avoid reevaluation of their life situation or to escape having to face truths about themselves that are more easily suppressed. They promote crises and stress in order to feel something that will confirm they are alive—and coincidentally that will let them receive sympathy and attention from others. Adventuresome people appear to thrive on their "adrenaline rush," unaware of the damage they are doing to their bodies. They could be called "stress junkies."

The stress chemicals coursing through a stress junkie's body provide the punch needed to skip breakfast, work fourteen hours, and then throw a dinner party for twelve of their closest friends. They may be perfectionists who take on too much work (and they often work with other stress junkies). Their days of using the "high" of stress as a mood-altering device are numbered, but addictive.

Living this way for a sustained length of time puts a woman right on the edge and frequently results in pent-up, unresolved anger and frustration. A day of reckoning inevitably comes. The bottom falls out (or burns out). She finds she can't get out of bed in the morning, or she spends her coffee break hidden in the office broom closet, shedding uncontrollable tears.

Sometimes coming to terms with stress requires burning out like that, because it forces a woman to take a good honest look at herself, rather than rushing off to tackle more tasks. Admonitions to "be calm" are likely to create more stress for the effort. It is OK to say, "This is a problem that I must have the courage to look at and take baby steps to change."

Simple nurture

Women typically use nurturing and friendships to lower their stress. For women, the "fight-or-flight" stress response is not the only one. It seems that the hormone oxytocin, which is enhanced by estrogen in women and reduced by testosterone in men, encourages women to tend to children and gather with other women when stressed.[1] This response, called "tending and befriending," stimulates an increased release of oxytocin, which produces a calming effect. This unique feminine response has been overlooked because 90 percent of all studies on stress have been done on men. Apparently a woman's social ties may be a factor in reducing stress risks, and it helps explain why women tend to live longer than men. One study found that over a nine-year period, the women who had the most friends cut their risk of early death by more than 60 percent. A review of the Harvard Medical School Nurses' Health Study confirmed that women who had the most friends as they aged had fewer physical impairments and thus more reason to live a joyful life.

De-stress to avoid distress

To de-stress, don't forget about exercise, because it is such a huge stress alleviator; it helps to bring down high levels of cortisol and increases endorphins and serotonin, which inhibit the stress response. Exercising at least five days a week, and taking stress-diffusing breaks throughout the day will work wonders. Take the dog for a walk, breathe out stress, and breathe in with gratitude.

Pay attention to good nutrition. Eliminate refined sugars and carbohydrates, and eat four to five servings of fruit and vegetables and three servings of whole grains daily. This will keep you energized and less apt to "stress-eat."

Recognize the mental aspect of stress management: stress is not stress unless you perceive it as stress. It is how you react and act that will determine if it will be detrimental to your health. When you realize that stress can drive up blood pressure, increase your risk for stroke, raise cortisol levels, change your body composition, increase your risk for degenerative disease, and rob you of energy and zest for life, you will be motivated to de-stress by using whatever combination of techniques works for your unique situation.

Anger

Angry outbursts are common in some households, especially at certain times of the month.

PMS mood symptoms include irritability and frustration at the least, and in that week or two before menstruation, many women suddenly find themselves weeping or screaming with anger or feeling unusually tense with no real cause in their external circumstances. Their hormonal fluctuation has resulted in a lowered level of the brain chemical neurotransmitter serotonin.

A woman can feel completely out of control. One minute she's preparing dinner and the next minute she's ranting and raving at her children.

Lifestyle changes could be in order. She needs to take back the mastery over her emotions. The apostle Paul was not a woman, of course, but he understood how this works:

> Do you not know that all those who run in a race run, but one receives the prize? So run, that you may obtain it. Everyone who strives for the prize exercises self-control in all things. Now they do it to obtain a corruptible crown, but we an incorruptible one. So, therefore, I run, not with uncertainty. So I

fight, not as one who beats the air. But I bring and keep my body under subjection, lest when preaching to others I myself should be disqualified.

—1 Corinthians 9:24–27

A stressed woman doesn't have to run a race—she can walk. Exercise should be part of any lifestyle change, and brisk walks should be part of every week. She can take a twenty- to thirty-minute walk every other day. Or she can try another type of fresh air exercise that she enjoys at least three to four times a week, such as riding a bike. Regular exercise can make all the difference in the world when battling hormonal imbalance. It helps to keep your metabolism high, which prevents weight gain, and it melts away stress. Walking is probably the safest exercise of all. It does not require expensive training, special equipment, instructional videos, computer programs, or special manuals. It doesn't require prior training or conditioning, and it doesn't require a great deal of physical exertion in the beginning. Walking is more natural than sitting, standing, or running, and it is not as stressful to the body as other forms of exercise. Walking eases back pains, slims the waist, lowers blood pressure, reduces levels of bad cholesterol, reduces heart attack risk, enhances stamina and energy, lessens anxiety and tension, improves muscle tone, is easy on the joints, reduces the appetite, increases aerobic capacity, can be done in short bouts, slows down osteoporosis and bone loss, and can be done even when traveling!

You may be thinking, "I've tried many exercise programs, but I never hang in there long enough to get results. I always quit too soon." Here's a tip: choose an exercise activity that you truly enjoy and make it a vital part of your day. Too many people get into trouble when they save exercising for their spare time. If you wait until you get around to it, you probably never will. Schedule exercise during the day as you would schedule an appointment—and do not break that appointment. Your exercise doesn't have to be structured. Look for simple opportunities to move a little more—park farther from your destination for a longer walk, take the stairs instead of the elevator, and toss a ball with your children or grandchildren in the backyard.

A lifestyle that includes friends, family, work, play, love, time for self, and time for spiritual growth leads to a well-rounded life that is balanced physically, emotionally, and spiritually. A woman can make her friends and family part of her exercise routine, if they are willing to do so. Exercise helps with disordered moods of all sorts. Not only does it moderate a woman's stress-filled anxiety and anger, it also helps with depression.

Depression

The many and varied symptoms of depression may include:

- Profound, persistent sadness
- Profound, persistent irritability
- Unexplained crying
- Loss of self-esteem
- Feelings of hopelessness
- Feelings of pessimism
- Feelings of helplessness
- Feelings of worthlessness
- Feelings of guilt
- Feelings of emptiness
- Continual mulling over the past, reviewing errors you have made
- Changes in sleeping patterns
- Changes in eating habits
- Unexplained weight gain or loss
- Restlessness
- Fatigue
- A "slow-down" of physical movements
- Inability to concentrate
- Memory difficulties
- Difficulty making decisions
- Loss of interest in usually pleasurable activities
- Loss of interest in sex
- Unexplained headaches, upset stomach, or other physical problems that are not helped with standard treatment
- Thoughts of suicide or death
- Actual suicide attempts

There are different degrees of depression ranging from mild to severe. Treatments can range from electroconvulsive therapy (ECT) for intractable depression to therapy, drugs, and nutritional and lifestyle modification for ordinary depression. Medications have helped many people regain their sense of equilibrium, but these medications carry potentially serious side effects and their use must be carefully monitored.

Depression can also be a result of prolonged stress, which causes a deficiency of amino acids, resulting in a biochemical imbalance. Other nutritional deficiencies, nervous tension, poor diet, mononucleosis, hormone shifts, thyroid disorders, allergies, and serious physical disorders can also cause depression. Depression can take the form of anxiety, sadness, and eating disorders—resulting in weight loss, weight gain, sleep disturbances, and numerous other problems.

GREEN TEA

L-theanine is an amino acid found in green tea that produces tranquilizing effects in the brain. For centuries green tea has been used in the Orient for its calming, curative properties without drowsiness. L-theanine increases GABA (gamma-aminobutyric acid), an important inhibitory neurotransmitter in the brain that helps regulate anxiety.

The common denominator for all types of depression is the neurotransmitter brain chemical known as serotonin. A decreased level of serotonin frequently causes depression, anxiety, and other symptoms. Hundreds of studies have shown that adding serotonin to the body can relieve the symptoms of depression and anxious depression, and it can help patients lose weight and normalize sleep patterns. Because it is not possible to give a person serotonin directly, the traditional medical approach has been to use a class of drugs known as SSRIs (selective serotonin reuptake inhibitors). These SSRIs prevent the reuptake of serotonin in the brain, which logically results in increased levels of serotonin.

In general the SSRIs are safe, and millions of prescriptions for them have been used. Drugs in this category include Prozac, Zoloft, Paxil, Celexa, Luvox, and others. As with any drug, there are side effects in certain individuals, but generally they are well tolerated. Rarely more serious problems occur in which patients experience unusual outbursts of temper and violence. Occasional episodes of nervousness and fatigue have also been observed.

Low serotonin levels are now implicated in a much wider variety of diseases than just depression. Some of these include sleep disorders, binge eating, attention deficit disorders, headaches, PMS, and food and carbohydrate cravings that commonly lead to obesity.

The body naturally converts certain chemicals—amino acids—to serotonin. Several chemicals fall into this category, but one that has aroused particular enthusiasm is an extract from the seed of a plant called *Griffonia simplicifolia*. This seed contains a chemical called 5-hydroxytryptophan (5-HTP), which helps to normalize the levels of the critical brain chemical serotonin. Usually the body uses an amino acid called L-tryptophan to convert to serotonin in the human body. Tryptophan occurs naturally in milk, turkey, and other foods. Before tryptophan is converted to the beneficial brain transmitter serotonin, it is first converted to 5-HTP. However, when 5-HTP is ingested directly as a supplement, 70 percent of it is converted to serotonin, compared to the 3–5 percent that comes from the tryptophan from foods.

5-HTP seems to help not only with depression but also with anxiety symptoms. Another benefit is that these neurotransmitter chemicals in the brain can have a direct effect on appetite, and 5-HTP can help overweight patients achieve weight loss. Insomnia, which is also common with depression, also decreases markedly when the patient is on this natural supplement.

5-HTP will often produce results when traditional prescription antidepressants fail. One study involved ninety-nine patients whose conditions did not respond to any attempts at alleviating their depression. They were given the supplement 5-HTP at dosages averaging 200 milligrams daily and ranging as high as 600 milligrams daily, and nearly half of them had a complete recovery. It would certainly make sense that if 5-HTP works so well in these hard-to-treat patients, it would work even better in the more commonly encountered mild to moderate depression. It not only works, but also the side effects are typically very mild, with the most frequent being mild nausea occurring in less than 10 percent of all patients. (However, because 5-HTP is eliminated through the kidneys, patients with renal disease should avoid 5-HTP, as should those patients with peptic ulcers.) For mild to moderate depression, a dose of 50 milligrams of 5-HTP three times daily for two weeks is a good starting level. The dosage can be increased to 100 milligrams three times daily if improvement is not seen. Coated capsules or tablets are now available, which seem to decrease the nausea that patients might experience.

Many types of recurrent chronic headaches (tension headaches, migraines) can be associated with serotonin imbalances. This knowledge has produced a new generation of prescription medications that affect serotonin receptors, such as Imitrex and Maxalt. Because of the effect of 5-HTP on serotonin, it could be added to this list.

It is common knowledge that low serotonin levels can lead to chronic sleep disorders. 5-HTP, in a dosage of 100–300 milligrams forty-five minutes before bedtime, has helped promote sleep by causing patients to go to sleep more quickly and stay asleep longer. It is wiser to start with the lower dose and gradually increase it after about three days. Since weight gain, headaches, and insomnia can indirectly cause depression in and of themselves, 5-HTP provides relief from these problems as well as improving the depression itself; therefore, it is very effective in fighting depression and anxiety.

Hugs for Emotional Health

You don't hear much about the importance of the simple sensation of touch—especially comforting, loving touch—where mood swings are concerned. Yet human touch may be the simplest solution of all, especially for women. Just as orphaned babies stop growing and thriving due to the lack of touch, we adults on some level do not thrive as well when our lives lack touch. Women especially respond to touch because their skin is more sensitive than a man's. Since women experience higher levels of stress and lower levels of the chemicals that combat stress, a woman's benefit of physical touch is powerful and necessary.

Simple touch can:

- Increase production of endorphins, DHEA, and growth hormone
- Lower the levels of stress hormones in your body
- Lengthen your life span
- Make your immune system stronger
- Lighten your mood and lessen your stress

Touching promotes elevated production of endorphins, DHEA, and growth hormone. The good news is that this can easily be achieved by hugging a loved one each day. Hugs can lower the levels of stress hormones and even lengthen life. Touching can make the immune system stronger and mood lighter. Touching, be it a hug, pat, or massage, provides many health benefits. A half-hour massage can boost a woman's immune system and lessen stress, making her feel calm and happier.

How can you incorporate more touch into your life?

- Kiss a friend hello on the cheek. Or give them a quick "hello" hug. These are quick anti-stress remedies.
- Consider buying a pet. Persons who give and receive love to and from their pets can satisfy their daily touch quota. Pets are often used in nursing homes to bring comfort to residents.

- Snuggle with your children while watching television. Tackle them for fun, and even give them a back rub. Touching your children can help them develop into loving, caring, and expressive adults.

- Rub your partner's back and neck for thirty minutes, then suggest that turnabout is fair play.

- After a long, steamy shower, get out your favorite aromatic lotion and give yourself a massage.

Western society has developed a "hands off" mentality. And yet the skin that our Creator gave us is the largest sense organ in our bodies and responds positively to every loving touch. If you do not have anyone to whom you can turn to for a soothing word or gentle touch, surround yourself with enjoyable textures around you. Velvety pillows, silky clothes, and smooth grass are all sensations we experience through the sense of touch. Take time today to explore creative ways to make your environment a more "touching" place to be. Soon your mood swings will be a thing of the past.

Chapter 7

HEART DISEASE

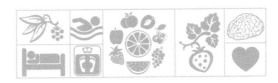

IF YOU WERE to ask women what they are most likely to die from, many would say breast cancer is their biggest fear. Some worry about ovarian cancer or colon cancer. The truth is, in women over the age of sixty-five, the number one killer is heart disease. In fact, in that age group heart disease claims more lives than all cancers combined. Women are five times more likely to die of heart disease than of breast cancer.[1]

Heart Attacks

Two of the most frightening words that a person can hear are the words "heart attack." For years doctors had believed that an artery was like a water pipe, which slowly collected plaque over the years, causing a buildup that eventually blocked the artery and caused a heart attack. It certainly seemed to be a logical explanation. Unfortunately it was wrong.

The arteries that are 90 percent blocked, we are learning, are *not* the arteries that cause most heart attacks! People with blocked arteries often experience angina, which is defined as chest pain on exertion. It is difficult for the blood to flow through their arteries when they exert themselves. But in heart attacks, more often there is a sudden onset of chest pain that begins in the middle of the chest and radiates outward, frequently through the left side and down the left arm. What is happening is that fatty plaque develops not just within the artery itself, but also in the wall of the artery. This plaque, which is covered by the lining of the arterial wall, builds up and actually causes the lining of the artery to rupture. When that happens, suddenly, the fatty material within the wall begins to protrude into the blood flow in the artery.

Because our bodies were created to repair themselves, when they detect any breach, such as the arterial rupture, the body's healing process signals a blood clot to form. In this case the effects of that natural healing process can be disastrous. Platelets begin to stick together, a clot begins to form, and in a period of a few minutes, that clot fills up the artery, blocking blood flow. In addition, the artery itself begins to constrict in order to stop the flow of blood from the breach in the wall's lining—again, with disastrous consequences. The result is myocardial infarction—a heart attack.

This disease that leads to a heart attack is known as atherosclerosis. Is there anything we can do to stop this process, or is it just "in our genes," an inevitable part of aging?

If a parent or sibling had early heart disease, and if you are obese, a smoker, or have other risk factors, ask your doctor about getting a cardiac CT scan to assess your real risk.

Atherosclerosis (also called hardening of the arteries) is really an inflammation in the arteries. When the LDL (bad) cholesterol forms a solid or semi-solid plaque or deposit that can stiffen artery walls, this plaque consists of white blood cells, smooth muscle cells, platelets, and other components, but it basically represents an inflammatory process in the plaque. There are at least four approaches you can take to help prevent this deadly problem from attacking your body.

Take low-dose aspirin. Amazingly half of the people with these artery-clogging plaques have normal cholesterol levels. It is the initial damage to the artery lining caused by the bad cholesterol that sets the stage for inflammation. This is why one low-dose (81 milligrams) "enteric-coated" baby aspirin can work wonders in preventing heart disease—it stops the inflammation. (The term *enteric-coated* should appear on the label of the bottle.) Interestingly regular aspirin (325 milligrams) may not be as effective as the low-dose aspirin.

TEA CAN SAVE YOUR LIFE

Tea is the most consumed drink in the world. Asian cultures have recognized a medicinal component for generations. Tea is rich in antioxidants (polyphenols and flavonoids), and research has verified its cancer-protectiveness and its ability to lower the risk of heart disease.[2] Tea also provides a relaxation effect due to a neurologically active amino acid, L-theanine, found almost exclusively in tea plants.

Take antioxidants. Why does the cholesterol damage the arteries? Damage is caused by the oxidation or breakdown of the LDL cholesterol, which enables it to harm the healthy cells lining the arteries. This is why it is so critical to provide antioxidants in the form of vitamin E (800 international units daily), vitamin C (2,000 milligrams daily), selenium (200 micrograms daily) along with others, such as the carotenes and coenzyme Q_{10}.

Lower homocysteine levels. Protein is another potential culprit in the development of atherosclerosis. It is not the protein we eat (which is good for us), but the breakdown of certain types of protein (amino acids) into a by-product known as homocysteine that can cause problems. High homocysteine levels can damage the arteries, and these levels increase when we lack sufficient amounts of B vitamins in our diet.

To keep homocysteine levels low and thus offer sufficient protection against hardening of the arteries, take 600 micrograms of folic acid daily, 75 milligrams of vitamin B_6 daily and 100 micrograms of vitamin B_{12} daily.

Policosanol. Policosanol is a chemical derived from sugarcane that has been found effective in reducing cholesterol levels. To prevent atherosclerosis, the LDL (bad) levels of cholesterol need to be under 130, and the HDL (good) levels of cholesterol should be well above 40.

GOOD FATS

Replace animal fats with good fat sources such as cold-water fish (salmon, mackerel, tuna, herring, crab, etc.), avocados, raw nuts, nut butters, seeds, and good oils such as olive, flaxseed, sunflower, and pumpkinseed.

Women and Their Hearts

Women are more likely to die of a heart attack than men. They are less likely to make it to the hospital for treatment, and even when they do make it, they are less likely to be diagnosed properly. Health care providers and women themselves often minimize their symptoms. It is important to be evaluated immediately if you experience any of the following symptoms: pain or discomfort in the center of the chest, neck, jaw, or left arm; shortness of breath; breaking out in a sweat; feeling faint or woozy; or indigestion.

For both women and men, the most common sign of a heart attack is pain or discomfort in the center of the chest. The pain or discomfort can be mild or strong. It can last more than a few minutes, or it can go away and come back. Women are more likely than men to have the "other" common signs of a heart attack. These include shortness of breath, nausea or vomiting, breathlessness, or perspiration. Some have a feeling of ominous doom, or pain in the back, neck, or jaw. The signs of a heart attack can happen suddenly. But they can also develop slowly, over hours, days, and even weeks before a heart attack occurs. A third of the time a woman's heart attack goes unnoticed.

The more heart attack signs that you have, the more likely it is that you are having a heart attack. Also, if you've already had a heart attack, your symptoms may not be the same for another one. Even if you're not sure you're having a heart attack, you should still seek medical help.

BOTANICALS/SUPPLEMENTS AND YOUR HEART	
Intervention	Benefit
Fish oils (omega-3)	First supplement ever recommended by the American Heart Association because of its ability to reduce cardio events.
Flaxseed	Provides positive lipid profile.
Nuts, particularly almonds, eaten daily	Improves blood lipids, homocysteine, and nitric oxide ratio.
Vitamin E	Take 400 international units vitamin E and 50 milligrams vitamin C twice daily. Foods high in antioxidants are highly recommended.
Tea and cocoa	Contain antioxidants and flavonoids.
Calcium	Improves HDL and LDL ratios.
Magnesium and potassium	Lower blood pressure and prevent irregular heartbeat.
Folate/folic acid and/or 5-formyltetrahydrofolate (5-FTHF) and 5-methyltetrahydrofolate (5-MTHF)	Lowers homocysteine, which injures cells that line blood vessels, and promotes coagulation; homocysteine is an independent risk factor for congestive heart failure in adults without prior heart attack.
Hawthorn leaf and flower extract (*Crataegus oxyacantha*)	Lower blood pressure, reduce angina, decrease progression of atherosclerosis.
Garlic (*Allium sativa*)	Lipid modulation; reduces hypertension; antioxidant properties.
Purified policosanols	Natural support for maintaining healthy blood lipid levels and platelets while promoting overall vascular health.
Coenzyme Q_{10}	Vital to cellular energy production; highly concentrated in the heart and other high-energy-requiring organs; antioxidant prevents LDL oxidation.

Heart Disease in Women

Among women between the ages of forty-five and sixty-four, one woman in nine will develop heart disease, but over the age of sixty-five, that number triples to one in three, which is what makes it the number one killer of women. Women are protected hormonally from heart disease in their younger years, but by the time they reach their sixties, they have caught up with men in the risk of developing heart problems.

"Heart disease" is more appropriately called cardiovascular disease (CVD). The cardiovascular system is the system in your body that circulates blood, carrying life-giving oxygen to and poisonous waste products from your vital organs. The word *cardiovascular* means "pertaining to the heart and the blood vessels." Therefore, cardiovascular disease is any disease that would affect those areas of the body. Cardiovascular disease often strikes suddenly and without warning. One in every two Americans dies of cardiovascular disease. (That's 50 percent!) Since 1984 the number of CVD deaths for females has exceeded those for males, with over 400,000 per year.[3] This crisis affects us all, whether we are facing it in our own bodies or watching it happen to someone we love. But the good news is that it is possible to prevent and even reverse cardiovascular disease before it becomes deadly.

Cardiovascular disease involves more than just heart attacks. It encompasses a host of ailments that affect the heart, blood vessels, veins, and arteries. Many of these ailments can affect your health without your even being aware of them.

GREEN TEA

Drinking one cup of green tea per day makes blood vessel walls more elastic and better able to expand to allow a free flow of blood, which can significantly lower a person's risk of developing heart disease or suffering a stroke.

Women tend not to acknowledge heart disease as their primary health risk and fail to institute changes that might reduce risk. Few who smoke are quitting, and obesity is hitting new records, with about 25 percent of women undertaking no regular physical activity. Over half of all women over fifty-five have high blood pressure, and 40 percent have elevated cholesterol. A woman with diabetes is as likely to die from a heart attack as a woman who has already had one. Those with Syndrome X (35-plus-inch waist, high fat in blood, poor cholesterol levels, high blood pressure) are at significant risk.

Reducing Heart Risk

Preventive strategies such as lowering the LDL (bad) cholesterol, strengthening the arterial walls, preventing platelets from clotting, and removing saturated fat from your diet can go a long way toward lowering your risk of a heart attack.

Saturated fats are mostly animal fats that are solid at room temperature. Plant-based saturated fats include liquid coconut, palm, and palm kernel oil. Saturated fat tells the liver to make artery-clogging LDL cholesterol. Eating too much saturated fat increases the risk of heart disease and other health problems.

Unsaturated fats are usually liquid and either polyunsaturated (safflower, corn, soybean, fish) or monounsaturated (olive, sesame, and peanut oils; almonds; avocados). Monounsaturated fats such as olive oil lower LDL and increase HDL, protecting against heart disease and benefiting the body in a number of other ways.

Consider this statement from the *Journal of the American Medical Association:* "Substantial evidence indicates that diets using nonhydrogenated unsaturated fats as the predominant form of dietary fat, whole grains as the main form of carbohydrate, an abundance of fruits and vegetables, and adequate omega-3 fatty acids can offer significant protection against CHD [cardiovascular heart disease]. Such diets, together with regular physical activity, avoidance of smoking and maintenance of a healthy body weight, may prevent the majority of cardiovascular disease in Western populations."[4] (Note that HRT is not mentioned as a heart-protective measure.)

Postmenopausal women can cut their risk of heart disease by up to 40 percent with thirty minutes of exercise daily (which can consist even of gardening and yard work).

Essential fatty acids (EFA), including omega-3, are essential because the body can't make them; they must come from food or supplements. They boost energy, reduce heart disease and pain from arthritis, and heighten immunity. Signs of depletion include fatigue, lack of endurance, dry skin and hair, and frequent colds.

Wonderful sources of omega-3 fatty acids include fish oils; fish; oils from flaxseed, borage, black currant, and primrose; sunflower seeds and pumpkin seeds. However, if you decide to have fish be your source of omega-3, you may risk ingesting excess mercury, a known environmental contaminant. A study in the *New England Journal of Medicine* reported a direct association between the risk of heart attacks and mercury levels.[5] If you are uncertain about the origin of your fish, a better choice may be to take capsules that come with proof they are mercury-free.

Mitigating Other Risk Factors

There is no avoiding the truth that the majority of cardiovascular disease can be attributed to lifestyle choices. Clearly, what you eat, your weight, and how much you move around is vital. Excess weight increases the burden on the heart. A sedentary person has twice the risk of someone who takes a thirty-minute stroll or works in her garden each day. Improvements in heart health are related to the amount of activity and not to the intensity of exercise or improvement in fitness.[6]

Exercise also has the benefit of helping people stop smoking; this is significant because up to one-fifth of all cardiovascular deaths are due to smoking.

Although some believe that alcohol in moderation (only one drink per day) protects against heart disease, more than one alcoholic drink a day elevates blood pressure and triglycerides. This is a particular threat to women. Of most concern is the 41 percent increase in breast cancer in women with two to five drinks per day (9 percent in women with less than one drink per day).[7] Because women have more fatty tissue than men, which contains less water than muscle, there is less body water available to dilute alcohol. Additionally, women metabolize alcohol differently. The key gastric enzyme that degrades alcohol is lower in women than in men, allowing more alcohol to pass through the stomach and enter the blood. To make matters worse, women are more vulnerable to liver disease, and if they have an alcohol problem, they are more likely to develop a quickly deteriorating alcoholic hepatitis and cirrhosis of the liver. They are also more susceptible to alcohol-related cardiomyopathy, a weakening of the heart muscle.

Heart disease is a preventable disease with modifiable risk factors. To sum up, having high blood pressure, diabetes, high cholesterol; smoking; and being sedentary and overweight all increase your risk of developing heart disease.

SALT

Salt is one of your body's most important minerals along with potassium. It helps regulate your cell's water balance. Yet too much of it can cause fluid retention and breast tenderness, and it can increase your risk of hypertension (high blood pressure) and heart disease.

Women with low blood pressure can benefit greatly by adding ⅛ teaspoon of sea salt to an 8-ounce glass of water every morning to help increase blood volume.

Most women, however, consume too much salt. As salt substitutes, try fresh herbs, garlic, and lemon to season your foods and enhance the flavors.

Cholesterol

Having some cholesterol in your body is natural and healthy. It serves important functions such as making cell membranes and some hormones. When it is found in high levels, however, it can lead to heart attacks or strokes. Remember that there are two types of cholesterol—LDL ("bad" cholesterol) and HDL ("good" cholesterol). LDL, or low-density lipoprotein, is responsible for delivering cholesterol to the body; high levels of LDL can clog arteries, thus increasing your risk of having a heart attack or stroke. HDL, or high-density lipoprotein, carries cholesterol away from the bloodstream; having high levels of HDL actually reduces your risk for heart disease.

Women who are forty-five or older should have their cholesterol checked. To be accurate, your blood should be drawn after you have fasted. If you have a family history of high cholesterol or other risk factors for heart disease, you may need your cholesterol checked earlier. Total cholesterol less than 200 is ideal. Between 200 and 239 is borderline high, and 240 or more is high. As discussed above, it is important to know the breakdown between good and bad cholesterol. Your LDL should be under 130. If it is between 130 and 159, it is borderline high, and if it is 160 or more, it is too high. HDL greater than 60 helps to lower your risk of heart disease, whereas if it is less than 40, your risk increases. Having high triglycerides (a form of fat made in the body) usually accompanies high cholesterol. Elevated triglycerides are usually due to obesity, lack of physical activity, smoking, and a diet rich in carbohydrates.

The first step to lowering your cholesterol is changing your lifestyle. This can be very difficult to do, but it can make a dramatic impact on your health. Stop smoking, follow a low-fat diet, limit your alcohol intake, and get regular exercise. If you attempt these changes for six months to one year without good results, or if your cholesterol is too high to be changed through these efforts alone, your doctor may place you on a cholesterol-lowering medication. (This must not replace your efforts, because continuing to follow a healthy lifestyle is important.)

If your figure looks more like an apple than a classic hourglass, you need to know that you are at greater risk for heart disease (and diabetes). You can find body mass index (BMI) calculators on the Internet[8] to calculate your body mass index, a number that categorizes your weight as overweight (25–29.9), obese (above 30) or underweight (18.5 or less). A healthy body mass index is between 18.5 and 24.9.

More Than Heart Attacks

The human heart is a strong muscle, used to pump blood through the arteries and veins, dispensing important nutrients and oxygen and carrying waste material away from the cells. There are four chambers in the heart. The two upper chambers—the atria—are smaller than the two lower chambers—the ventricles—the large pumping chambers that propel the blood out of the heart and throughout the body. The right ventricle pumps blood to the lungs; the left ventricle pumps blood to the rest of the body. A lot can go wrong with your heart besides heart attacks.

Arrhythmia: irregular heartbeats

Most people who experience arrhythmia don't go in to see their doctor and say, "I have an irregular heartbeat, Doc. I think I might have an arrhythmia." Many people aren't even aware that they are experiencing an arrhythmia. Their observations may be something like, "My heart has been doing flip-flops lately," or, "I've been having palpitations." Sometimes they may feel as if their heart has paused or skipped a beat, which can be quite frightening to people who don't understand what is happening to them. Some people may even begin to wonder if they are about to have a heart attack. If their heartbeat pauses for longer than a beat, they wonder if their heart will start to beat again!

NATURAL SUBSTANCES TO PREVENT OR REVERSE ARRHYTHMIA

It is best to combine these supplements in your regimen because their effect is synergistic, meaning their effectiveness multiplies when they are used together.

- Coenzyme Q_{10} (50 milligrams/day): Coenzyme Q_{10} helps to stabilize the normal rhythm of the heart.
- Magnesium (400 milligrams/day): For years magnesium was used in hospital IVs to help stabilize patients' heart rates.
- Omega-3 fatty acids (fish oil) (2,000 milligrams/day): Among its many benefits, fish oils help stabilize irregular heartbeats.
- Potassium (99 milligrams/day): Potassium levels that are either too high or too low will frequently cause irregular heart rates.
- Calcium (500 milligrams/day): Calcium can both stabilize heart rate and lower blood pressure.

Arrhythmia, or irregular heartbeat, is a very common condition. In fact, all of us have a type of irregular heartbeat called a sinus arrhythmia, which is quite normal. If you sit in a chair, resting and breathing at a normal pace, and you take your pulse, you might notice that your pulse does not beat at an entirely steady rate. It may speed up slightly and then slow back down. Heart rates often vary according to a person's breathing pattern or other changes that are occurring in the body. Becoming aware that this (sinus arrhythmia) is a normal occurrence will keep you from feeling alarmed. In fact, it is a good idea for you to become aware of the usual heart rate patterns that occur in your own body so that you can detect the more dangerous forms of arrhythmia that could occur in case of disease.

Bradycardia

One heart irregularity to which we must pay much closer attention is bradycardia. The root word *brady* means "slow," and *cardia*, of course, refers to the heart; therefore, bradycardia indicates that a person's heart is beating more slowly than it should.

How do you know how slow is too slow? You can start by getting to know your own body's heart rate. Athletes in peak physical condition will have slower heart rates than people who are not in shape. On the average if your resting heart rate drops to fifty beats per minute or lower, you could be experiencing bradycardia. If that is the case, you should get your heart rate checked by your doctor.

Your heart will keep beating even if there is a disruption of the electrical signals; the ventricles will contract on their own, continuing to send life-giving blood to your brain and other vital organs. It is a survival mechanism, designed to keep you alive. The problem is that the "emergency" contractions will only occur at about forty beats per minute. At that rate, you will notice that something is very wrong. Because there isn't enough blood circulating, you will become light-headed, dizzy, perhaps even disoriented. When this happens, it is time to seek medical attention. Bradycardia—slow heartbeat—can signal that there is a problem with this built-in pacemaker that God designed. If it is not kicking in correctly, your heart rate can drop dangerously low, and your vital organs—especially the brain—can experience a devastating lack of blood flow.

Tachycardia

At the opposite extreme from bradycardia is the condition of tachycardia, meaning a heart rate that is too rapid. The prefix *tachy* means "fast," and, again, *cardia* means "heart." Tachycardia is generally defined as a resting heart rate that is over one hundred beats per minute.

Tachycardia can be caused by a variety of conditions. One of the first things that doctors will check for is anemia, because some people with anemia will experience heart rates of up to one hundred twenty beats per minute. If you have a drop in your hemoglobin, which carries oxygen to your tissues and organs, you will start to experience a lack of oxygen in those tissues. God has designed the body to signal the heart to beat faster when this occurs so that more blood will be carried throughout the body in a shorter period of time. If you are experiencing an unusually high heart rate, ask your doctor to perform a simple blood test to determine whether or not you are anemic. It can tell you the levels of iron in your blood, the number of red blood cells, and so on.

Tachycardia can also be a symptom of an underlying infection somewhere in the body. On the average, for every degree of above-normal temperature (fever) in the body, the heart rate goes up ten beats per minute. So if your heart begins to beat faster on a consistent basis, begin to suspect that an infection may be lurking in your body of which you are unaware. Have your doctor perform a check of your white blood cell count to see if your body is fighting an infection.

Atrial fibrillation

A more dangerous form of irregular heartbeat is called atrial fibrillation. The term *atrial* refers to the upper chambers of the heart, and *fibrillation* means "a shaking or a quivering motion." Therefore, atrial fibrillation is a quivering that occurs in the upper chambers of the heart. A good comparison to what goes on would be that of the agitator in the washing machine that slaps the clothes around in the water to get them clean. However, when the atria of the heart begin to agitate in this manner, they aren't stirring up soap and water; they're affecting platelets that are in the blood-stream. When these platelets are stimulated in such a manner, they begin to stick together, forming the dangerous condition of a blood clot. The blood clot then finds its way into the ventricles of the heart, where it can be pumped into the carotid or verte-bral arteries, go straight to the brain, and cause a stroke.

Because atrial fibrillation can cause such a dangerous situation, it is important to have a checkup performed occasionally. Most people suffering from atrial fibrillation would not be able to feel it occurring in their chests. If the condition is diagnosed, there are several ways to treat it. The first course of action is to prevent the platelets in the blood from sticking together. For younger people (under the age of seventy), a simple daily dose of aspirin is effective. However, if a person is over the age of seventy, a blood thinner is usually required.

Sometimes atrial fibrillation can indicate a problem in one of the valves in the heart. Your doctor can perform an echocardiogram to check for this condition. If a valve is too narrow or has developed stenosis (thickening), the blood may not be passing through it correctly and may be disrupting the beating of the heart.

Premature ventricular contraction

All of us will experience premature ventricular contractions (PVCs) at one time or another, but it is when they become a consistent pattern that they become very dan-gerous. In a normal heartbeat, just before the electrical impulse is fired, there is an instant of time called "repolarization." It occurs just after the completion of one heart-beat, during which the heart is preparing to beat again. However, if the heart fires off too early, there will then be a long pause, and the ventricles of the heart begin to overfill with blood. This causes the ventricles to stretch and then beat strongly to push all of the blood into the bloodstream. You will notice this strong heartbeat and will often have to pause for breath or cough in order to recover.

Many times premature ventricular contraction can be caused by stress, too much caffeine, or even stimulants found in over-the-counter cold medicines that contain pseudoephedrine. Most of the time, the situation is benign. However, if there are three or more of this type of heartbeats that occur right in a row, something called ventricular tachycardia, or VT, occurs. When VT occurs, which involves several longer pauses in a row between heartbeats, there is no time for the heart to fill with blood. Suddenly there is a shortage of blood being pumped from the heart. People have been known to pass out at this point from the lack of circulation to their brains. Once this dangerous cycle has begun, the person may progress quickly from VT to a very serious problem called ventricular fibrillation.

Ventricular fibrillation is very different from atrial fibrillation because it affects the large pumping chambers of the heart. If these chambers begin to quiver, they are not pumping blood effectively, and the person will die very quickly if drastic measures—usually an electrical shock to the heart—are not taken.

HELP YOURSELF TO CHOCOLATE

Good chocolate is rich in antioxidant flavonoids called flavanols (procyanidins, epicatechins, catechins), known to lower the risk of heart disease, lung cancer, asthma, and diabetes. Some studies have shown benefits to HDL and LDL ratios, and for lowering clotting and keeping arteries flexible. This is good news for those who love chocolate—as long as it's the best. One ounce of high-quality, very dark chocolate has double the antioxidant punch of red wine or other chocolates.

Congestive heart failure

Congestive heart failure occurs when there has been so much damage to the heart muscle that it cannot pump fast enough to prevent a buildup of fluid in the lungs. Many people with congestive heart failure also have swelling or edema in their ankles. These patients usually reach a point where their lung capacity is so limited that they cannot lie flat in bed because when they do, it is difficult to breathe. They also become out of breath quickly with any level of exertion.

Long before doctors understood what congestive heart failure was, they knew that a certain family of plants—the rose family, which includes hawthorn extract—was helpful in strengthening the contractions of the heart. Today we are rediscovering the uses of this invaluable natural substance. Controlled studies have been conducted that show the benefits of hawthorn extract in the reversal of congestive heart failure. It has a direct effect on the electrical impulses of the heart, shortening the refractory time between heartbeats and allowing the heart to pump more fluid more effectively.

High blood pressure

High blood pressure (hypertension) is accurately called the silent killer. It is often the root cause of many other health problems, especially heart disease. As blood pressure readings approach 140/90 and above, a silent but deadly process begins weakening the body. Strain is placed on the heart muscle, and thickening in the pumping chamber of the heart (left ventricular hypertrophy) occurs. The incidence of heart attack and stroke begins to increase, and the kidneys begin suffering damage.

Many people believe that if their blood pressure is up, they will have some visible sign such as headaches or nosebleeds—but these are the exception. Usually there is no warning of high blood pressure until something breaks. By then it is a major battle to overcome the problem.

As pressure and stress increase, damage is done to blood vessel walls leaving them susceptible to cholesterol buildup. When high blood pressure is coupled with elevated insulin levels (common with diabetes and obesity) heart disease is likely. Excess insulin, the response to high sugar levels in the blood, raises cholesterol and blood pressure.

Easy-to-read blood pressure measuring devices are readily available at most pharmacies or drug stores. Persistent high blood pressure is significant; a few sporadic high blood pressure measurements are not.

YOUR BLOOD PRESSURE

Blood pressure is made up of two measurements or numbers. The first number is the systolic blood pressure. This is the peak blood pressure when your heart is pumping out the blood. The second number is the diastolic blood pressure. It's the pressure your blood vessels feel when they are at rest between beats. A normal blood pressure is 120/80 or lower. High blood pressure is 140/90 or higher. If your blood pressure is between 120/80 and 140/90, you have something called "prehypertension."[9]

Three natural supplements, when taken on a daily basis, can lower blood pressure naturally and with no side effects.

Potassium. There are many studies that indicate the power of potassium to reduce blood pressure. Potassium effectively protects the kidneys also because of its role in protecting the lining of blood vessels from damage. Consuming five or more servings of fruits and vegetables daily is the ideal way to obtain sufficient potassium. Potassium can also be obtained in supplement form. Taking 99 milligrams daily will ensure constant blood levels, and your dietary intake of fruits and vegetables can simply build on this consistent level.

Polyphenols. Polyphenols are important compounds found in numerous foods. A particular association has been reported between certain polyphenols found in olive oil and the lowering of blood pressure. Other oils, such as polyunsaturated oils, do not have these polyphenols present and do not produce a reduction in blood pressure. The compounds contained in the olive oil stimulate the production of a natural substance, known as nitric oxide, already present in the human body. Nitric oxide is important because it tends to relax and dilate blood vessels, which results in blood pressure reduction. These phenols also function as antioxidants that reduce the damaging effects of free-radical compounds that can affect blood vessels.

It is interesting to note that olive oil is an important component of the Mediterranean diet. This may be one of many reasons that countries around the Mediterranean Sea have some of the lowest recorded rates of heart disease in the world.

Hawthorn berry (100–250 milligrams three times daily) protects the heart from free-radical damage and helps the heart pump blood efficiently.

Magnesium. Magnesium is an increasingly important mineral. People who consume higher-than-average amounts of magnesium in the form of fruits and vegetables have significantly lower blood pressure.

A study known as the Honolulu Heart Study, showed that magnesium was the most consistent substance that correlated with lowering the systolic and diastolic (upper and lower) blood pressure. This study consistently showed that the lower the blood magnesium levels, the higher the risk of heart attacks and the development of high blood pressure.[10] Low magnesium levels also correlated with hardening of the arteries and the accumulation of cholesterol plaque in the carotid arteries, which supply blood to the brain. With magnesium supplementation, both the systolic and diastolic blood pressures fall, because magnesium causes blood vessels to dilate. Magnesium can also help prevent heart palpitations and improve cholesterol levels. Even greater benefits are noted when the magnesium is taken with a potassium supplement and when salt is restricted in the diet.

Over the past several decades, the dietary intake of magnesium in the United States has decreased by slightly over 50 percent. At the same time, we are facing an epidemic of high blood pressure, with more Americans than ever being diagnosed with hypertension.

YES TO BANANAS!

Bananas can actually function as blood-pressure-lowering agents because they are high in potassium, which can lower blood pressure. They also contain a natural compound used in our most popular antihypertensive medications. One of the most popular classes of antihypertensives (blood pressure medications) is known as ACE inhibitors or ACE blockers, and this class of drugs has also shown a protective effect on the kidneys of diabetics. Studies indicate that bananas contain a natural ACE blocker and can lower blood pressure up to 10 percent in patients who consume two bananas daily.[11]

Because high blood pressure can creep up slowly on a person, giving no warning signs until it is too late, it is so important to be proactive in preventing potential serious problems before they strike. Have your blood pressure checked regularly. If your doctor sees readings in the 130/80 range, it is time to take action. You should lose weight, exercise, increase your consumption of fruit—especially bananas—and consider taking supplements that can lower blood pressure, including garlic capsules (the equivalent of one clove daily).

If your readings are found to be consistently over 140/90, you may need to be on a one-pill-a-day prescription drug such as one of the ACE drugs. Once you start taking a drug, this does not mean that you will be on it for life. When lifestyle changes are made, many patients can decrease and even go off their blood pressure medicine. However, this must be done with close monitoring under the care of a physician.

Balancing Your Blood Pressure

Hypertension (high blood pressure) is ranked in stages:

	Systolic	Diastolic
Normal	120	80
Stage I	140 to 159	90 to 99
Stage II	160 to 179	100 to 109

	Systolic	Diastolic
Stage III	180 to 209	110 to 119
Stage IV	210 or higher	120 or higher

Even Stage I hypertension can cause serious health problems, increasing your chances of stroke, heart attack, kidney failure, and more.

Follow these dietary guidelines:

- Eat a high-fiber diet.

- Reduce salt consumption, including salty foods such as cured, smoked foods, soy sauce, potato chips, and dry soup mixes. Salt promotes fluid retention, which increases blood pressure.

- Avoid caffeine; it raises blood pressure.

- Add garlic, celery, olive oil, and flaxseed oil to your diet.

- Avoid soy sauce, MSG, and canned vegetables.

- Avoid smoked and aged cheeses and meats, chocolate, canned broths, and animal fats.

- Limit sugar intake. It can increase sodium retention.

- Avoid phenylalanine (found in diet foods and drinks) and antihistamines.

The good news is that you can, in most cases, lower your blood pressure by losing weight and making lifestyle changes, which would include an exercise program, and you can head off developing heart disease for years to come.

Chapter 8

BREAST CANCER AND OTHER WOMEN'S CANCERS

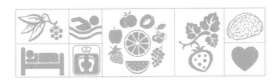

D EVELOPING BREAST CANCER is perhaps a woman's greatest fear. And it is a valid concern, as one in eight (12 percent) of women in the United States will contract breast cancer in their lifetime, regardless of family history. In 2014 about 232,670 women were diagnosed with breast cancer, and about 40,000 of them will die from the disease.[1] When detected early, the five-year survival exceeds 95 percent.

KEY STATISTICS ABOUT BREAST CANCER

Breast cancer is the most common cancer among American women, except for skin cancers. The American Cancer Society's most recent estimates for breast cancer in the United States:

- About 231,840 new cases of invasive breast cancer will be diagnosed in women.
- About 60,290 new cases of carcinoma in situ (CIS) will be diagnosed (CIS is non-invasive and is the earliest form of breast cancer).
- More than 40,000 women will die from breast cancer.[2]

Breast cancer occurs when a tumor (abnormal growth of cells) begins in the breast and grows without control. It usually begins in the milk ducts that line the breast, but it can also start in the lobules, or glands that make breast milk. Lymph vessels drain the breast into lymph nodes under the arm, under the neck, and in the chest wall. If the cancer in the breast reaches these lymph nodes and continues to grow, swelling will occur. The cancer can then spread beyond the breast into other tissues of the body.

It should be noted that the majority of breast lumps are not cancerous. Although all breast lumps need medical evaluation, many are harmless. The most common cause of breast lumps is fibrocystic breast disease, which is characterized by cysts and a thickening of the milk glands. Symptoms include lumpiness in the breast and tenderness that becomes more pronounced just before the menstrual cycle. This condition typically affects women between the ages of thirty and fifty because this is when there is a higher incidence of hormonal fluctuations and imbalances, primarily estrogen dominance, which seems to "feed" cysts or multiply their occurrence. As a rule benign lumps are usually tender and moveable while cancerous lumps are usually painless and do not move freely.

There are four basic types of breast lumps:

1. *Lipoma*—a benign, painless tumor made up of fatty tissue. Usually considered harmless, it has the potential to become malignant.

2. *Fibroadenoma*—commonly found in women twenty years old and older. It is usually a rubbery, firm, and painless mass commonly found on the upper portion of the breast.

3. *Cystosarcoma*—a fast-growing benign tumor that grows in the connective tissue of the breast. In rare instances it can become malignant.

4. *Carcinoma of the breast*—a dimpled area of skin can be seen directly over the lump; can also include a dark discharge from the nipple. Malignant breast lumps are usually the size of a pea and are hard to the touch. In 90 percent of cases, only one breast is affected at a time.

> The National Cancer Society website www.cancer.gov/bcrisktool/ contains the Breast Cancer Risk assessment tool, which can be used to help you identify your own personal risk of developing breast cancer.

Options for Treatment

If breast cancer is detected, there are various options for treatment. You may be a candidate for a lumpectomy, or removal of the tumor mass itself. When the entire breast needs to be removed, it is called a mastectomy. There are different types of mastectomy, including the following: simple mastectomy, partial mastectomy, modified radical mastectomy, and radical mastectomy. In addition to surgery, chemotherapy and/or radiation may be recommended by your doctor.

After undergoing treatment for cancer, it is important to take care of yourself and to undergo recommended follow-up tests and exams. Breast cancer can recur, but many more women are diagnosed with breast cancer than actually die as a result of it. This indicates that breast cancer is curable, especially if caught early.

Risk Factors

While the cause of breast cancer is unknown, there are certain risk factors that predispose a person to developing breast cancer. Just because you have a risk factor does not mean that you will develop the disease, and many women without any risk factors will develop breast cancer. The following factors have been associated with an increased risk of developing breast cancer:

- Gender: Being a woman is the single biggest risk factor for developing breast cancer. However, contrary to popular belief, men can develop breast cancer.

- Age: The risk of developing breast cancer increases with age, with 79 percent of new cases and 88 percent of breast cancer deaths occurring in women over fifty.[3]

- Family history: If you have a close relative with breast cancer, defined as a parent, sibling, or offspring, your risk doubles.

- Genetic mutations: Carrying a gene that predisposes you to breast cancer makes it likely that you will develop the disease.

- Personal history of breast cancer: If you have already developed breast cancer in one breast, you are more likely to get it again in the other breast.

- Race: Caucasian women are more likely to develop breast cancer.

- Previous breast biopsy: An abnormal breast biopsy in the past puts you at a higher risk of breast cancer.

- Previous radiation exposure: Undergoing treatment to the chest with radiation raises your risk of breast cancer.

- Prolonged menstrual cycles: Having periods beginning before age twelve or lasting past age fifty-five increases your risk.

- DES (diethylstilbestrol) exposure: If your mother took diethylstilbestrol when she was pregnant with you, then you are at an increased risk.

- Not having children: If you do not have children or you have your first child after age thirty, your risk is increased.

- Hormone replacement therapy: HRT can increase your risk of developing breast cancer if taken for several years. It does not appear that estrogen replacement alone increases this risk. However, if you have had breast cancer, you should not take estrogen, as it may increase your chance of recurrence.

- Alcohol: Drinking even one drink daily increases your risk.

- Obesity: Being overweight increases your risk of developing breast cancer.

Genetic testing. Until recently, testing for genes that increased one's chance for breast cancer was somewhat of a no-win proposition. If you found you were a carrier, there was nothing you could do. Today early intervention and a number of options are possible for high-risk situations. Sometimes just knowing one has a propensity for disease becomes motivation to follow good health practices.

HRT REDUCTION RESULTS

After increasing for more than two decades, female breast cancer incidence rates began decreasing in 2000, then dropped by about 7 percent from 2002 to 2003. This large decrease was thought to be due to the decline in use of hormone therapy after menopause that occurred after the results of the Women's Health Initiative were published in 2002. This study linked the use of hormone therapy to an increased risk of breast cancer and heart diseases. Incidence rates have been stable in recent years.[4]

How to Decrease Your Risk of Breast Cancer

The following factors have been associated with a decreased risk of breast cancer:[5]

- Weight loss: Losing eleven pounds or more can decrease risk, especially among postmenopausal women.

- Physical activity: Studies show that exercising (at least thirty minutes on five or more days of the week) may reduce your risk by 30 to 40 percent.

- Limited alcohol consumption: The more alcohol you drink, the greater your risk. Limit yourself to no more than one drink per day—12 ounces of beer, 5 ounces of wine, or 1.5 ounces of liquor.

- Breastfeeding: Breastfeeding for at least four months offers women some protection against breast cancer.

- Avoiding cigarette smoke: Smoking is responsible for 30 percent of all cancer deaths.

- Bypassing HRT: HRT increases the risk of breast cancer and heart disease. Talk to your doctor about the risks and benefits.

The National Cancer Institute has estimated that simply making changes in dietary intake might prevent 60 to 70 percent of breast cancer cases. Here are some ideas:

Eat that tofu! The incidence of breast cancer in Asia and other parts of the world is very low. Researchers believe the low rates of breast cancer are due, in large part, to the intake of natural, fermented, non-GMO, organic soy products. More recently, as Asians have begun following a Western-type diet, their incidence of breast cancer has risen steadily. The phytoestrogens, known as isoflavones, in soy are actually cancer preventives. These isoflavones bind to estrogen receptor sites and guard against the development of breast cancer. Soy contains other natural chemicals such as protease inhibitors, which prevent cancer-promoting genes from being activated, and saponins, which can keep cancer cells from multiplying. Do avoid the highly processed soy products such as soy milk, soy protein substitutes, and soy fats such as soybean oil as new research shows they may have adverse effects on health. Enjoy moderate amounts of miso, tempeh, natto, tofu, or soy sauce.

Take red clover extract. Perhaps an even better source of these beneficial isoflavones is an extract derived from red clover. Red clover contains four major isoflavones that, when taken daily, appear to be a promising and effective method for women to protect their bodies against the potential of breast cancer.

Eat lots of fish. Study after study demonstrates that women who eat more fish have lower rates of breast cancer. Part of this protection comes from omega-3 fatty acids that are found in fish such as salmon, cod, mackerel, herring, sardines, and trout. The omega-3 fatty acids are really oils that the human body can convert to a chemical known as prostaglandins. Certain types of protective prostaglandins keep breast cells from multiplying and dividing. Patients with a strong family history of breast cancer or unusually thick breasts with increased amounts of fibrous tissue might want to consider taking omega-3 capsules daily. A study published in the *Journal of the National Cancer Institute* found that taking fish oil capsules increased the concentration of omega-3 fatty acids (EPA and DHA) in breast tissue. Some other natural sources are walnuts and flaxseed.

Limit saturated fats. Most saturated fats come from animal sources (meat and dairy sources). Avoid fatty meats in particular, including poultry cooked with the skin on. Also avoid milk fat, including butter and cheese. Animal fats harbor toxins and pesticides, which only increase the cancer risk of the person who consumes them unless you choose organic varieties. Some plant-based oils, such as palm oil, palm kernel oil, and coconut oil, also contain primarily saturated fats, and hydrogenated vegetable oils (transfatty acids) have been declared unsafe at any level. (Transfatty acids are used in foods to help them maintain taste and last while they sit on a shelf for an indefinite amount of time.) Look for "partially hydrogenated oil," on the label, including in products claiming to be fat free or "cholesterol free." Also, consume sparingly the polyunsaturated vegetable oils such as flax/linseed, rapeseed/canola, soybean, cottonseed, sunflower seed, corn, and safflower oil, because they contain omega-6 fatty acids, which may actually promote breast cancer.

Add kiwi fruit to your diet. The *Journal of the American College of Nutrition* ranked kiwi fruit as the most nutrient-dense of all fruits, providing vitamin E, magnesium, and potassium, and also proving to be a good source of dietary fiber. Kiwi provides twice as much vitamin C as an orange, and studies show that vitamin C can inhibit breast cell division, thus reducing the risk of breast cancer.

Eat ten almonds and five prunes a day. Nuts (better if salt-free) are a rich source of vitamin E, they also play an important role in preventing breast cancer. Laboratory studies show that vitamin E decreases the incidence of mammary tumors that form after exposure to cancer-causing substances. It actually prevented the cancer cells from developing and provided a killing effect on the cells after they developed. Combine your almonds with prunes for extra benefits. Prunes have turned out to be a medical "super fruit" in the fight against cancer. Because of the prune's remarkable ability to absorb oxygen-free radicals, they may also help retard the aging process in the body, especially in the brain.

Go orange. There are some unique chemicals contained in citrus fruits, and especially in oranges, that fight breast cancer. *Hesperetin* and *naringenin* both prevent cancer cell division and also help neutralize cancer-causing chemicals in the body. Another chemical found in oranges, *limonene,* has potent cancer-fighting properties.

Fiber, fiber, fiber. Fibers tend to bind cancer-causing agents in the gastrointestinal tract and keep them from being absorbed. If you cannot get enough fiber in the form of fruits, vegetables, beans, and whole-grain flours, you can supplement your diet with psyllium fiber. Remember that the most fiber is contained in the skin or peel of the fruit or vegetable. Caution to those who have wheat or gluten sensitivities: try organic, sprouted whole grains or choose gluten-free whole grains such as brown rice, oats, buckwheat, amaranth, millet and quinoa.

Eat cabbage, broccoli, and brussels sprouts. A unique chemical compound in cruciferous vegetables called indole-3-carbinol (see below) reduces the body's production of certain types of estrogen leading to breast cancer. Cruciferous vegetables include kale, cauliflower, turnips, collard greens, and more.

Eat your carrots. Beta carotene is the best source of vitamin A, and supplements can supply what your food does not. Studies consistently show that populations that consume the most vitamin A have the lowest levels of breast cancer.

Speaking of soy…

The phytoestrogen molecules in natural soy looks much like human estrogen. They are classified into three groups and vary in their activity:

1. *Isoflavones* (genistin/genistein, daidzin/daidzein, glycitin/glycitein, formononetin, biochanin A), found in soy and garbanzo beans and other legumes (tempeh, soy, miso, tofu, kudzu root, red clover), are hormonal regulators, weak estrogen mimics, antiestrogen, antioxidant, and anticancer interventions. The amounts and ratios of actives vary from plant to plant.

2. *Lignans* are found in the cell walls of plants and are made bioavailable by the action of intestinal bacteria on grains (flaxseed, whole cereals such as rye and wheat berries, brans, and soybeans). They are hormonally active and known for their anticancer activity.

3. *Coumestans* are not a major natural source of phytoestrogens for humans (clover, sunflower seeds, and bean sprouts).

Most American women consume less than 3 milligrams of isoflavones per day compared to Asian women, whose soy-based diet contains 40–80 milligrams per day. Higher isoflavone intake increases sex-hormone-binding globulin and, in conjunction with other chemical processes, lowers estrogen production.[6] This is particularly true in populations that have used them for a lifetime and less certain for those who increase their intake at a later age. Still, further research suggests that consumption of as little as 10 milligrams per day may be associated with health benefits.[7] The genistein in soy increases the activity of dopamine and other neurotransmitters helpful for depression. Soy foods are generally recommended over highly concentrated soy pills, especially for cancer patients, because supplement production changes the effect. However, women are not always good about adding tofu and such to their diet. It really does not matter whether you consume fermented soy foods, such as tempeh, or nonfermented, such as tofu, because fermentation occurs through the action of gut bacteria. Genistin and daidzin are more prevalent in nonfermented soy. What counts in the soybean concentrate you purchase, fermented or nonfermented, is the actual amount of isoflavones on the label—verified by independent third-party analysis.

Supplemental indole-3-carbinol. Indoles are phytochemicals (substances derived from plants) that may negate the effects of circulating bad estrogen to prevent further growth of breast tumors.[8]

Indole-3-carbinol (I3C), which is derived from cruciferous vegetables, may inhibit estrogen metabolites that are associated with breast and endometrial cancer. It is a powerful antioxidant that protects DNA and makes cells resistant to damage. Studies have shown that this vegetable extract may stop human cancer cells from growing by 54–61 percent and may even provoke cancerous cells to self-destruct (a phenomenon known as *apoptosis*). I3C also protects against dioxin, an environmental carcinogen. For breast cancer health I3C works to help modulate estrogen metabolism. In addition it increases the conversion of estradiol to the weaker estrogen, with a 50 percent reduction within one week. Under laboratory conditions it inhibited the growth of MCF7 breast cancer cells better than Tamoxifen. I3C is activated by stomach acid, so do not take it with antacids. A 200 milligram capsule can be taken twice daily.

> *For more information on breast cancer and awareness, visit the Susan G. Komen for the Cure Web site at ww5.komen.org.*

Breast Cancer Detection

Breast cancer can be detected through screening techniques, such as mammography, clinical breast exams, and self breast exams. Some signs to look for are: swelling in a part of the breast, skin irritation or dimpling, nipple pain or inversion, redness or scaliness of the breast skin, discharge other than a milky substance, or a lump under the arm. If something suspicious is found through screening, diagnostic tests will be performed through an ultrasound and MRI. Suspicious areas or lumps may need a biopsy to obtain a sample of the tissue to see if it is cancerous or not.

DIAGNOSTIC METHODS FOR BREAST CANCER INCLUDE:

- Mammography
- Needle aspiration
- Ultrasound
- Thermographic screening
- Surgical biopsy

Breast self-examination

Women should perform self-exams on a regular basis to evaluate for lumps or other abnormalities. Breast self-examination can be accomplished either standing up or lying down. Some women do it in the shower as a way of developing a routine. How, when, or where it is done is not nearly as important as simply doing a self-exam.

If a woman does not become familiar with the feel and consistency of her own breasts, she will not be able to distinguish a change in them, which can be the first sign of disease. Women who rely only on their annual gynecologic exam to screen for breast disease leave themselves vulnerable the rest of the year. The woman who regularly examines herself is in much better position to notice a change compared to the physician who sees her only once a year. (This applies not only to the breast exam but also to other areas such as mole surveillance to prevent skin cancer.)

The breast exam is done with two fingers pressing the breast tissue against the rib cage or gently squeezing between the fingers. This allows for the detection of irregular tissue or lumps. Most of these will be fibrous cysts or benign tumors, but it is important to enlist the patient to ensure there is no change in size between visits. Abnormalities detected during the breast exam may require evaluation with sonography or mammography to exclude breast cancer.

Mammography

Mammograms are one of the best methods for early detection, yet millions of women in the United States age forty or older have never had a mammogram. There are many reasons for this, such as cost, access to health care, ignorance about risk, and fear of discomfort or radiation exposure. The American Cancer Society recommends yearly mammograms beginning at age forty to help detect breast cancer. If you have a family history of breast cancer in a first-degree relative, you may need to start sooner because you are at risk for breast cancer. However, you do not need to have a family history of cancer or an abnormal breast exam to undergo mammography. Mammography is a good way to detect breast cancer in an early stage; however, it will not detect all breast cancers.

> In a fifteen-year study involving 250,000 fifty-five to seventy-year-old women, mammography reduced breast cancer deaths by 21 percent compared to the control group.[9]

A mammogram is an X-ray of the breast tissue used to detect abnormalities in both symptomatic and asymptomatic women. Mammography was initially developed in 1969, though X-rays have been used to examine the breasts for over ninety years. Since then there have been great technological advances, even in the last twenty years. One change is the amount of radiation delivered during the exam. The machine used to image the breasts produces lower energy X-rays with less tissue penetration than a normal X-ray.

A screening mammogram takes images of two views of your breasts, which are then displayed for a radiologist to read. Digital mammography captures the images electronically, giving the radiologist the advantage of changing the contrast or magnifying the image on a computer to better evaluate certain areas. This helps to more accurately identify cancer in women under the age of fifty and in those with dense breasts. The entire procedure takes about twenty minutes. It is important to have your mammograms done at the same imaging center each year if possible, so that previous images can be compared. Having a computer read the images serves as a second opinion to double check the radiologist. This can pick up some cancers that the doctor might have missed, but it can also lead to unnecessary biopsies.

> Most health insurance programs, including Medicare and Medicaid, cover the cost of mammograms. Low-cost mammograms are available in some communities. You can contact the American Cancer Society for information about facilities in your area.
>
> In addition, the National Breast and Cervical Cancer early Detection Program (NBCCeDP) provides breast and cervical cancer early detection testing to women without health insurance for free or at very little cost. To learn more about this program, please contact the Centers for Disease Control and Prevention (CDC) at 800-232-4636 or www.cdc .gov/cancer/nbccedp/.

If an abnormality is detected, it does not necessarily mean that you have cancer. Only about 10 percent of women who undergo screening mammography will have to undergo additional tests because of an abnormality. These tests include a follow-up mammogram, often with magnification views; a breast ultrasound; or a magnetic resonance imaging (MRI). And of the women who undergo additional screening, only a handful will be diagnosed with breast cancer. Some special situations require other tests as well. If you or your doctor notices a lump or mass, you will need a diagnostic mammogram as opposed to a screening mammogram. This test takes more pictures as well as magnification views to evaluate the suspicious area. An ultrasound may also be performed to provide more information about the abnormal area. If you have breast implants, additional images are taken as the implant is pushed back into the chest while the breast tissue is pulled forward. If you are at high risk for developing breast cancer, your doctor may order an MRI in addition to a screening mammogram.

Other devices can be used, such as nuclear medicine scans, thermal scans, laser scans, and electrical scans. Computerized Thermal Imaging (CTI) picks up increased heat radiated by cancer cells and differentiates between normal and suspicious spots, thus reducing the number of biopsies. Ductal lavage is FDA approved and is much like a Pap test, seeking to collect cells "that are thinking about becoming cancer." Cells are extracted from the milk ducts. Ductal lavage is intended to be used in conjunction with mammograms. "Precancerous" cells give a woman a heads-up choice about preventive treatment. Needle biopsies make diagnosis much less invasive than before by aspirating a few cells into a syringe.

The problem with mammograms is not whether or not they are effective at detecting early evidence of breast cancer—they are. The controversy is over when a woman should start having them. There is no disagreement with beginning to have mammograms at age fifty. Those who do not recommend their use in forty- to forty-nine-year-olds maintain that "abnormal" growths subject women to invasive procedures for prevention they may have never needed. Those who recommend earlier mammograms maintain that women have smaller tumors, less chance of spread, and more breast conservation than those who wait. Insurance companies are increasingly paying for double reads, either by a second technician or a computer.

Although the number of cancer cases is increasing, the good news is that there is also a rising group of cancer survivors. This is because our knowledge of the disease has changed. Early detection has always been one factor in survival and proper treatment.

Simply by shifting your food choices even slightly in favor of more vegetables such as broccoli and brussel sprouts and fewer high-fat treats every day enlivens your body and protects you from cancer.

We now know that most cancers respond positively to diet improvement. You can help your body rebuild healthy cells while starving out cancer cells by avoiding "dead," heavily processed foods; refined sugars; excessive caffeine; food dyes; and pesticide-sprayed foods, which encourage cancerous cells to grow. Besides, diet improvement will boost the immune system in general. Cancer attacks when the immune response is low, whether from overwork, emotional upheaval, poor diet, or exposure to toxic substances. All of these factors change your body chemistry in a negative way, making it hard for your immune system to defend you from disease.

Cervical Cancer

Cancer of the cervix develops when normal cells in the lining of the cervix, where the innermost cells of the cervical canal connect with the cells on the surface of the cervix, become abnormal and develop changes that eventually turn into cancer.

Cervical cancer does not develop overnight. With proper screening, it can usually be caught and treated at an early or precancerous stage. Despite this, about 12,900 new cases of invasive cervical cancer will be diagnosed in the United States in 2015, and about 4,100 women will die from cervical cancer.[10]

Because of widespread use of the Pap smear test, the number of deaths from cervical cancer has dropped significantly in the last thirty years.[11] The majority of cases of cervical cancer diagnosed today are in women who have never had or not recently had a Pap smear. If an abnormality is found, it can almost always be treated before progressing to cancer. Therefore, it is important to undergo routine testing as recommended by your doctor and to have follow-up testing if an abnormality is found. If cancer is found early, it can be cured over 90 percent of the time.

If you receive a diagnosis of invasive cervical cancer, the treatment is hysterectomy (removal of the uterus and cervix) if caught early. More advanced cases are treated with radical hysterectomy (removal of the uterus, cervix, and surrounding tissue) or chemotherapy and radiation.

Most cases of cervical cancer are preventable. There are definitive risk factors that predispose you to develop cervical cancer. Infection with certain strains of human papilloma virus can lead to the development of cancer. If you have had a sexually transmitted disease in the past, your risk is greater, and if you were exposed to DES (diethylstilbestrol) before birth, you are also at greater risk. Precancerous lesions and early-stage cervical cancers do not produce any symptoms. They must be detected through routine screening.

Symptoms of invasive cervical cancer include abnormal bleeding or discharge and pain or bleeding during intercourse. Whether you are found to have a precancerous lesion or an invasive cancer, your doctor will recommend further workup and treatment. If an abnormality is detected with a Pap smear, your doctor will usually perform a colposcopy. This is a procedure where your doctor visualizes the abnormal area on your cervix with binoculars and takes a biopsy for further testing to see if dysplasia (a precancerous condition) is present. The tissue is then graded as "mild dysplasia," "moderate dysplasia," or "severe dysplasia." Most cases of mild dysplasia will not progress to cancer, while moderate or severe cases have a higher risk of becoming cancerous. Your doctor may recommend a procedure to remove these abnormal cells so that they do not progress to cancer.

Uterine Cancer

The most common type of uterine cancer is endometrial cancer, which starts in the lining of the uterus, or endometrium. It is the fourth most common cancer in women, behind lung, breast, and colon cancers.[12] If caught early and confined to the uterus, it is effectively treated with a hysterectomy.

Endometrial cancer is most common in women who are postmenopausal, though it can be found in younger women on occasion. It is usually caught early because most women develop symptoms of vaginal bleeding either between periods or after menopause.

If endometrial cancer is found in the uterus, it can be treated with a surgical hysterectomy if caught early. Other treatments used if it is more advanced include progesterone therapy, chemotherapy, and radiation. Patients need to be followed closely after treatment for return of the cancer.

Endometrial cancer develops over a period of time. First, the cells that make up the lining of the uterus grow and proliferate in response to estrogen. They become abnormal and, if not treated, can grow out of control, becoming cancerous. Therefore, conditions that increase your exposure to estrogen increase your risk of developing endometrial cancer. Some of these conditions include the following:[13]

- Obesity: being overweight raises your risk two to four times. A higher level of fat tissue increases your level of estrogen.
- Age: more than 95 percent of uterine cancers occur in women 40 and older.
- Eating a diet high in fat.
- Estrogen replacement therapy (ERT) without progesterone if you have a uterus. (Unopposed estrogen causes the lining of the uterus to grow, while progestins cause the lining to shed.)
- Personal/family history of uterine, ovarian, or colon cancer. This may be a sign of Lynch syndrome (hereditary nonpolyposis colorectal cancer or HNPCC).
- Ovarian diseases, such as polycystic ovarian syndrome (PCOS), which cause irregular ovulation and irregular menstrual cycles.
- Diabetes (frequently associated with being overweight).
- Never having been pregnant.
- Number of menstrual cycles (periods): if you started having periods before twelve years old or went through menopause late, your risk of uterine cancer may be higher.
- Pelvic radiation to treat other kinds of cancer. The main risk factor for uterine sarcoma is a history of high-dose radiation therapy in the pelvic area.

- Tamoxifen use. This breast cancer drug can stimulate the lining of the uterus to grow and cause cancer in one out of every five hundred women who take it.

Contact your doctor if you develop irregular vaginal bleeding, bleeding at times other than when you have your period, or bleeding after you go through menopause. He or she may want to perform an exam and special tests such as a Pap smear, biopsy, or ultrasound. If cancer is suspected or further testing is needed, you may need to undergo a D&C (dilation and curettage: dilation of the cervix and surgical scraping out of the lining/contents of the uterus).

Ovarian Cancer

Ovarian cancer is epithelial cancer, which means it starts on the surface of the ovary and spreads throughout the pelvis and abdomen. It usually progresses to an advanced stage before it is diagnosed. In 2014 it was estimated that 21,980 women would be diagnosed with ovarian cancer, and 14,270 would die from it.[14]

Symptoms of ovarian cancer can be vague, making it difficult to diagnose at an early stage. Some of the symptoms include the following:[15]

- Pain or swelling in the abdomen.
- Pain in the pelvis.
- Gastrointestinal problems, such as gas, bloating, or constipation.

If you have these symptoms for three weeks or more, you should contact your doctor. A pelvic exam and ultrasound can be used to detect ovarian cancer. A blood test called a CA-125 can also be ordered if cancer is suspected. If any of these tests show suspicion for cancer, your doctor may refer you to a women's cancer specialist (gynecologic oncologist) for staging and treatment.

Surgery for ovarian cancer consists of the removal of the affected ovary or both ovaries and any additional tissue or organs that it has spread to. If the cancer has spread beyond the ovaries, treatment also consists of chemotherapy and, rarely, radiation.

After diagnosis and treatment of ovarian cancer, your doctor will monitor you closely for recurrence of the disease. The likelihood of recurrence depends on the stage of diagnosis, with early stage cancers having a survival rate of 90 percent for five years or more, with most being cured.[16] However, most ovarian cancers are diagnosed at an advanced stage.

> ## HEALTH ALERT
>
> Several studies have indicated that women who use talcum powder in the vaginal area after bathing have a 60 percent increased risk of ovarian cancer. Women using genital powder deodorant sprays have a 90 percent increased risk.[17] These products are to be avoided.

Avoid and Conquer the Big C

"Proactive" is the key word in the war against women's cancers. Follow a healthy lifestyle, pay attention to changes in one's body, and schedule regular screenings. Ideally you will never get cancer at all!

Chapter 9

OSTEOPOROSIS

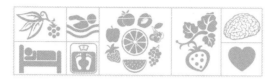

MOST PEOPLE PICTURE their bones as a skeleton with hard, dried bones. However, only 75 percent of your skeleton is made of a strong, compact bone called cortical bone. This is the main type of bones in your arms, legs, and ribs.[1] It regenerates slowly at about 2 to 3 percent per year.[2] Your remaining bone mass is trabecular bone, a spongy, porous, and lightweight bone with many holes in it. This type of bone is found mainly in the pelvis, hips, and spine, and it regenerates much faster than cortical bone[3] at approximately 25 percent a year.[4] Also, trabecular bone is more prone to osteoporosis.

During the early growth years new bone formation dominates, and very little bone is resorbed into the body. From the end of puberty to about age thirty-five, the body maintains a good balance of bone formation and bone resorption. However, after age thirty-five the process of dissolving the bone becomes increasingly dominant. After forty it actually accelerates, and after menopause, usually around age fifty, it increases even more.

Put another way, bone mass usually reaches its peak when a woman is about thirty-five years old. Between the ages of fifty-five to seventy, women typically experience a 30 to 40 percent loss of bone mass.[5] Realize that over your life span, if you are a woman, you will lose approximately 50 percent of your trabecular bone and 30 percent of your cortical bone.

Women and Osteoporosis

Osteoporosis, in which bones become porous and brittle, can happen to men as well as women, but it is most well-known as a women's disease associated with menopause. Under osteoporosis conditions bone turns over at an increased rate, with bone resorption exceeding new bone formation. The bone mineral density is decreased, by definition, 2.5 standard deviations below that of the peak bone mass of a normal healthy twenty-year-old. This condition affects four to six million women.[6]

WHEN SHOULD WOMEN BE
SCREENED FOR OSTEOPOROSIS?

The International Society of Densitometry and the National Osteoporosis Foundation have very similar recommendations about when to have a bone density test. Their recommendations for bone density tests include the following:

- Women who are 65 years of age and older
- Postmenopausal women under age 65 with risk factors such as smoking, weighing less than 125 pounds, and a family history of osteoporosis
- Women with a history of a low-trauma fracture (hip, wrist, or spinal fracture from minor trauma)
- Women with a health condition associated with low bone density or bone loss (hyperthyroidism, hyperparathyroidism, rheumatoid arthritis, vitamin D deficiency, etc.)
- Women taking medications associated with low bone density or bone loss (thyroid hormone medications, seizure medications, excessive doses of corticosteroids, medications that block sex hormone production, etc.)
- Women being treated with drugs for osteoporosis or being recommended for treatment due to evidence of bone loss
- Women whose standard skeletal X-rays show reduced bone density
- Women should be screened for osteopenia starting at age fifty.[7]

Statistics concerning osteoporosis are alarming. By the time half of all women reach the age of sixty, osteoporosis becomes evident on their X-rays. By the time a woman reaches eighty years of age, she can easily have lost almost half of her bone mass and not even be aware of it! The most frequent clue that alerts a woman to the fact that she has osteoporosis is a fracture of some sort, perhaps a broken hip or a broken leg. Many times a woman may think she was injured as the result of a fall, but what happens in many cases is that the fall is actually the result of the injury. A woman may be walking along, and because her bones have become so ravaged by the disease, a bone will break, and that is what actually causes her fall. In the United States there are approximately 1.5 million fractures per year due to osteoporosis.[8]

Risk factors for developing osteoporosis include the following: age over sixty-five, Caucasian race, low weight or low body mass index, history of fracture, family history

RISK FACTORS FOR OSTEOPOROSIS

You are at an increased risk of developing osteoporosis if you have any of the following risk factors. Notice that some risk factors are uncontrollable, such as your gender, ethnicity, and family history. Others are very much under your control, such as your intake of certain nutrients, smoking, and excessive drinking.

- Blonde or redheaded with fair skin
- Caucasian and Asian
- Thin (weighing less than 125 pounds)
- Short stature and small bones
- Postmenopausal
- Never been pregnant
- History of anorexia nervosa, bulimia, or early menopause
- Family history of osteoporosis
- Inactivity (a sedentary lifestyle)
- Smoking or excessive alcohol consumption (more than one drink a day for women)
- Excessive physical exercise
- Excessive stress or depression
- Hyperthyroidism
- Hyperparathyroidism
- High homocysteine level
- Have had a gastric or small bowel resection
- Long-term use of corticosteroids (such as prednisone), thyroid medications, and Lupron, which is a medication for endometriosis
- Long-term use of anticoagulant medication such as heparin, which is a blood thinner
- Long-term use of certain anticonvulsants
- High vitamin A intake
- High animal protein intake
- High sugar intake
- High sodium intake
- Excessive intake of sodas containing phosphoric acid (most have it)
- Low calcium intake
- Nutritional deficiencies

of osteoporosis, cigarette smoking, lack of estrogen replacement or early menopause, lack of exercise, poor nutrition, and diet low in calcium. Certain medical conditions and medications also increase the risk of osteoporosis.

The Bone Renewal Process

To prevent and overcome osteoporosis, you first need to understand how your bones mature, develop, and then begin to lose mass in midlife. Your bones are composed of approximately 70 percent mineral salts and 30 percent protein matrix.[9] The protein matrix is mainly composed of collagen fibers, chondroitin sulfates, and hyaluronic acid.

Calcium salts are the most essential element of bone formation, and 99 percent of the calcium in your body is stored in your bones. Only about 1 percent of your total calcium is in your blood and inside your cells.[10]

Calcium phosphate is a mineral salt that is present in the protein matrix and provides strength to the bone. The calcium and phosphate form crystals that are bound to the proteins and are arranged in an orderly pattern and called hydroxyapatite.

To understand this better, imagine a sidewalk made of iron rebar. The iron rebar is like the cross-links of proteins of collagen, and the concrete surrounding the rebar is similar to the hydroxyapatite crystals composed of mainly calcium and phosphorus. Concrete without rebar is not nearly as strong as concrete with rebar, and it is the same with our bones. They must have this strong collagen protein as well as hydroxyapatite surrounding them.

Many people think that once our bones are formed, they remain the same forever. However, our bones are made of living tissue that is continually being renewed throughout our lives. There are two main types of bone cells: osteoclasts and osteoblasts. Osteoblasts are cells that build bone and make hydroxyapatite in collagen. The osteoclasts are always searching for older bone that needs to be renewed. These cells break down the old bone using enzymes to dissolve collagen as well as hydroxyapatite. They leave behind very small lesions. The osteoblasts then move into these small spaces and produce new bone. Therefore, old bone is being dissolved continuously, and new bone is being formed. This renewal process is called "remodeling." The status of our bones is actually dependent upon the delicate balance of these two processes.

As we age, our bodies (particularly our bones) absorb calcium with less and less efficiency. A child usually absorbs 50 to 70 percent of the calcium from his or her food. However, adults may absorb only about 20 to 30 percent of the calcium in their diets, and older adults absorb even less calcium.[11] As you grow older, this lack of calcium is the single most important factor contributing to the decrease of bone mass and the increased risk of chronic osteoporosis. To understand osteoporosis, it's important to realize how much your body needs this vital nutrient.

OSTEOPOROSIS			
Why?	How?	Who?	Results?
The exact condition of your bones can be calculated. Osteoporosis risk increases the first five years after periods stop. This is a preventable disease in most cases.	The gold standard is a DXA (Dual X-ray Absorptiometry). Wrist and heel bone screening can be used to see if a DXA is necessary.	Menopausal women; family history; history of an eating disorder; low calcium ingestion as teen; steroid use (for arthritis or asthma); lack of or extreme exercise (marathon runner, ballet dancer); all women by age sixty-five; earlier for white or Asian women with one risk factor; any midlife or older woman who breaks a bone.	The DXA compares your results with other women your age and against younger women.

The Role of Hormones

Sex hormones are produced primarily by the ovaries and testes, and as we age, our bodies produce fewer and fewer of them. The rapid decrease of the hormone estrogen in women's bodies during menopause puts them at a greater risk of developing osteoporosis than men, whose hormone levels decrease much more gradually with age. There is a direct relationship between the lack of estrogen during and after menopause and the development of osteoporosis. Low progesterone levels may also be associated with bone loss, especially in premenopausal females.

Warning Signs

When bone mass in women begins to decrease after about age thirty-five most women do not realize it is happening because bone loss occurs without symptoms. But the osteoporosis that develops as a result of significant bone loss does have several telltale symptoms. They typically occur when the disease has reached an advanced stage and include the following:

Fractures. This is the wake-up call that most often alerts people that they have developed osteoporosis. Among healthy people, fractures only happen when a serious trauma to the bone has occurred, but in people with osteoporosis fractures can occur after minor traumas, such as bending over, lifting light objects, coughing, sneezing, bumping into a piece of furniture, or stepping off a curb. Fractures of the rib, compression fractures of the spine, and fractures of the hip are the most common fractures experienced by those with osteoporosis. (Compression fractures of the spine can pinch the spinal nerves, creating chronic pain and eventually leading to hip fractures and fractures of other bones throughout the body.) Also, it is common for people with osteoporosis who break one bone to have recurring fractures of the same bone or to break other bones as well.

Any fracture in a person with osteoporosis is serious because bones that are not as dense as they should be do not heal quickly, and sometimes they don't heal completely. But hip fractures are especially serious. They can lead to loss of independence, loss of function, and death.

HIP FRACTURES

The majority of hip fractures happen to people over age sixty, and because women are more prone to osteoporosis than men are, they experience the majority of these hip fractures—roughly 70 percent of them. In 2010 there were more than 250,000 hospitalizations for hip fracture. Some estimate this number could reach 290,000 by the year 2030.[12]

Pain. Persistent pain in the spine or muscles of the lower back, chronic discomfort or pain in the neck that is not caused by an injury, or pain in the hip are common symptoms of osteoporosis. Nighttime leg cramps and aching or tenderness of the bones are also symptoms.

Loss of height. Some people notice that their clothing doesn't fit the same or that their pants are too long but still don't make the connection to loss of height as a result of bone loss. You can keep track of your height if you get annual checkups. Be sure your doctor keeps a chart on your height, measured without shoes.

Dowager's hump or worsening scoliosis. A dowager's hump is an actual hump that develops due to the progressive curvature of the upper back and neck. Stooped posture and back pain can accompany these warning signs.

Compressed organs. As a consequence of compression fractures of the spine, the abdominal organs can become compressed, leading to an enlarging belly, constipation, and weight loss. People may become short-waisted and appear to have a belly or increased folds of skin on their abdomen as compression fractures occur.

Shortness of breath. Because of compression fractures of the thoracic spine, patients may develop shortness of breath since the lungs are not able to fully expand.

Dental problems. Other signs of osteoporosis include periodontal disease and loss of teeth as osteoporosis affects the jawbone.

Osteopenia and Early Detection of Osteoporosis

You don't have to wait until you are experiencing the symptoms above to start monitoring and improving your bone health. Osteoporosis is a progressive disease, and the earlier it is detected, the easier it is to stop and reverse.

Before osteoporosis develops, there is a stage called osteopenia, which is defined as having bone density that is lower than average but not low enough to be diagnosed as osteoporosis. It is natural to experience some level of low bone density (osteopenia) as you age, because old bone breaks down faster than new bone is made. But it is possible to slow this progression into osteoporosis and even stop and reverse it.

The best way to arm yourself is prevention. If you are young, follow the recommendations below to make your bones as strong as possible now. This will make it less likely that you will experience significant bone loss when you are older. The next best defense against osteopenia and osteoporosis is early detection. Whether or not you are experiencing any symptoms, if you have any of the risk factors, ask your doctor about a bone density test.

Diagnosing osteoporosis

Standard skeletal X-rays do not always help detect osteoporosis, because bone loss is not visible on an X-ray until you have lost more than 30 percent of your bone mass.[13] Therefore, special tests that use radiology to measure the density of minerals such as calcium in your bones have been developed. Bone mineral density (BMD) testing helps your doctor estimate the strength of your bones and predict your chances of experiencing a fracture or other symptom of osteoporosis.

The DEXA scan (dual-energy X-ray absorptiometry) is the most accurate of all bone mineral density tests and therefore is considered the gold standard. Since there may be differences in the bone mineral density in different areas of the body, most doctors request at least two sites be measured. Sites that are most commonly tested include the hips, spine, and forearm, with the areas of greatest concern being the hips and spine.

Other tests that measure BMD are peripheral dual-energy X-ray absorptiometry (P-DEXA), dual photon absorptiometry (DPA), ultrasound, and quantitative computed tomography (QCT). These tests vary in accuracy, cost, and levels of radiation exposure.

After you undergo testing, your bone mineral density is compared to average young adults of the same gender and ethnicity. The difference between your BMD and the average BMD is expressed as a standard deviation (or SD). The SD is your T-score and is either a positive or negative number. The World Health Organization defines osteoporosis as having a T-score of 2.5 or more standard deviations below the average (in other words, a T-score of -2.5 or less).[14] Osteopenia is defined when the T-score is between 1 and 2.5 standard deviations below average (a score of -1 to -2.5). A normal bone density receives a T-score of one standard deviation or less below the average (a score of 0 to -1). If you have osteopenia, your doctor will probably want to check your DEXA scan approximately every two years.

BONE DENSITY T-SCORES

T-Score	Condition
0.0 to -1.0	Normal bone density
-1.0 to -2.5	Osteopenia
-2.5 and lower	Osteoporosis

Osteoporosis screening

Screening should be performed in all women age sixty-five and older, and in post-menopausal women under age sixty-five if they have a risk factor. It should not be repeated more frequently than every two years, unless new risk factors develop or treatment is initiated.

Bone density is measured by comparing the results to that of a young healthy woman at her peak bone mass. The difference is measured in standard deviations and is translated into a T-score. A T-score between -1.0 and -2.5 is designated as low bone mass, or osteopenia. If left untreated, it could progress to osteoporosis. Osteoporosis is defined as a T-score -2.5 and lower. Sustaining a fracture due to a fall from standing height or less also makes the diagnosis of osteoporosis.

EASY TEST

It is not difficult to determine your risk for osteoporosis. The DXA test (Dual X-ray Absorptiometry) releases minimal radiation, takes less than twenty minutes, and doesn't require that you remove your clothes!

A variety of medications are available for prevention and treatment of osteoporosis. The most fundamental of them is calcium supplementation. The National Institute of Health recommends daily calcium supplementation with 1,000 milligrams for pre-menopausal women ages twenty-five to fifty and postmenopausal women who are younger than sixty-five and are on estrogen replacement therapy. Women over sixty-five, or postmenopausal women not on estrogen, are recommended to take 1,500 milligrams daily. Vitamin D (produced from sunshine on the skin) is also important to aid in calcium absorption; 400–800 international units is the recommended daily dose.

Despite its other contraindications (notably increased breast cancer), hormone replacement therapy has been shown to decrease the risk of osteoporotic fracture. Estrogen has been proven to halt the progression of osteoporosis and even reverse the disease, especially when it is combined with calcium and vitamin D.

AGING SKIN AND VITAMIN D

As you age, changes in your skin's structure will reduce your ability to convert vitamin D to its active form by up to 60 percent by the time you reach age sixty-five.[15]

In addition to estrogen, a class of medications known as selective estrogen receptor modulators (SERMs) work to reduce fractures without increasing the risk of breast cancer. Bisphosphonates are medications that work to reduce bone resorption and bone loss. Parathyroid hormone and calcitonin both act to increase bone formation and are options for treatment.

How to Get Enough Calcium

We all know that calcium is needed for strong, healthy bones, but how much calcium do you need every day?

HOW MUCH CALCIUM DO I NEED?[16]

The amount of calcium you need each day depends on your age. Average daily recommended amounts are listed below:

Life Stage	Recommended Amount
Children 9–18 years	1,300 milligrams
Adults 19–50 years	1,000 milligrams
Adult women 51 and up	1,200 milligrams

Dairy products are an excellent source of calcium. An 8-ounce glass of milk (that's just one cup) contains about 300 milligrams of calcium. It's interesting to note that the fat content of the milk does not change the amount of calcium. In other words, you get the same amount of calcium (300 milligrams) from any 8-ounce glass of milk: fat-free, low-fat, skim, whole, or lactose-free. Most other dairy products, such as yogurt, cheese, kefir, and buttermilk, also contain high amounts of calcium. You don't have to limit yourself to cow's milk and products made from it; goat's milk and yogurt, cheese, and kefir, are also good sources of calcium. Organic versions of the products are best.

Unfortunately some women are allergic to dairy products or are lactose intolerant, and they will need to consume other dietary sources of calcium. Small amounts of calcium are found in many foods, but there are only a few foods that contain large quantities of this vital mineral. Vegetables such as broccoli, cauliflower, peas, and beans are high in calcium. In addition, nuts—including Brazil nuts, hazelnuts, and almonds—and seeds, such as sunflower seeds, contain high amounts of calcium.

NONDAIRY FOODS WITH THE HIGHEST AMOUNTS OF CALCIUM	
Sardines, canned in oil, with bones	3 ounces contain 324 milligrams
Salmon, pink, canned, solids with bone	3 ounces contain 181 milligrams
Spinach, cooked	½ cup contains 120 milligrams
Turnip greens, boiled	½ cup contains 99 milligrams
Kale, cooked	1 cup contains about 94 milligrams
Kale, raw	1 cup contains about 90 milligrams
Chinese cabbage, raw	1 cup contains about 74 milligrams
Broccoli, raw	½ cup contains 21 milligrams
Bread, whole-wheat	1 slice contains 20 milligrams
Almonds	1 ounce (about 22 nuts) contains 75 milligrams of calcium

Which Calcium Supplement Is Best?

A confusing array of choices present themselves when you go to buy calcium supplements. You may find it useful to explore this topic in depth by doing a little online research. For the purposes of this book, we will talk about the two most commonly available forms of calcium supplements: calcium carbonate and calcium citrate.

Calcium carbonate is the most common calcium supplement on the market today. As a calcium salt it is very inexpensive as well as very convenient. A 1,000-milligram tablet of calcium carbonate contains 40 percent or 400 milligrams of elemental calcium, and it also contains 600 milligrams of the salt carbonate. So you are getting only 400 milligrams of elemental calcium in a 1,000-milligram tablet.

Another issue to be aware of is that calcium carbonate may be very poorly absorbed on its own, but when taken with food, studies have shown that absorption of calcium carbonate is about the same as calcium citrate, approximately 30 percent.[17] For that reason, it is best to take calcium carbonate with food.

However, without food, significantly less calcium is absorbed. That means if you take 1,200 milligrams of calcium carbonate a day, which is a typical dose, it translates to only 480 milligrams of elemental calcium a day. At best, you absorb only around 30 percent of that amount with food. So instead of getting 1,200 milligrams a day, you are actually only getting 144 milligrams of calcium a day.

Calcium citrate is the other very common calcium supplement that is sold over the counter and is better absorbed than calcium carbonate. However, the calcium content is actually lower than calcium carbonate. Calcium citrate contains 21 percent elemental calcium.[18]

So 1,000 milligrams of calcium citrate has only 210 milligrams of elemental calcium and 790 milligrams of citrate. Therefore, 1,200 milligrams of calcium citrate has only 252 milligrams of elemental calcium. Since approximately 30 percent is absorbed, that means only about 75 milligrams of elemental calcium is actually absorbed.

Calcium capsules usually dissolve better than calcium tablets. Calcium must dissolve in your stomach in order to be absorbed by your intestines. When you see "USP" on the label, you know that the calcium is pure and contains no lead or other toxic metals.

Many people have the idea that if calcium is dissolved in a liquid state, it is more easily absorbed. But this is not so because the majority of liquid calcium supplements out there are calcium carbonate, which is poorly absorbed (remember, only about 10 percent when taken without food and only about 30 percent when taken with food is absorbed). However, one benefit of a liquid calcium supplement is that it may be easier for the elderly to swallow.

What about coral calcium? Coral calcium has been advertised on TV for years. ConsumerLab.com, an independent testing lab, found that Coral Calcium Supreme had lead levels in excess of California standards for risk levels. There are similar lead dangers in oyster shell calcium, dolomite, and bone mill. The calcium found in coral calcium is in the calcium carbonate classification.

Keep in mind that solubility does not equal absorption. It is not accurate to conclude that because a certain form of calcium is more easily dissolved by your body it is automatically more easily absorbed. Remember also that if you do take a calcium carbonate supplement, it is best absorbed with meals since the calcium absorption depends on adequate hydrochloric acid produced by the stomach. When taking calcium supplements, divide up the doses during the day. Another reason for doing this is that your body can only absorb at most about 500 milligrams at a time.

> **Q:** If I take calcium supplements, does that completely eliminate my risk of bone loss?
>
> **A:** No! Many people—including many physicians—are under the wrong impression that if you simply take a calcium supplement, you will not lose bone or develop osteoporosis. That is simply not true.
>
> While calcium supplements are certainly a step in the right direction, the health of your bones depends on a number of different factors that affect your body's ability to absorb and utilize the calcium you consume. That's why it is important to implement all of the measures for healthy bones: proper diet, regular exercise, stress reduction, hormone therapy, and nutritional supplements.

Magnesium Too

Magnesium helps your body absorb calcium from your diet, and it also helps your bones to retain the calcium. Without enough magnesium, you are much more prone to lose bone rapidly. Magnesium is also necessary in order to prevent excess calcium intake from causing calcifications in soft tissues.

Foods highest in magnesium are nuts—such as almonds, walnuts, and cashews—whole grains, seafood, and legumes. Simply eat some extra nuts, whole grains, and legumes in order to add more magnesium to your bone-building program. Other magnesium-rich foods include:

- Apples
- Apricots
- Avocados
- Bananas
- Cantaloupe
- Grapefruit
- Soy (natural, organic)
- Brewer's yeast
- Brown rice
- Figs
- Garlic
- Kelp
- Lemons
- Lima beans
- Millet
- Peaches
- Black-eyed peas
- Salmon

Herbs that contain magnesium include alfalfa, bladder wrack, catnip, cayenne, chamomile, chickweed, dandelion, eyebright, fennel seed, hops, lemongrass, licorice, paprika, parsley, peppermint, raspberry leaf, red clover, sage, and yarrow.

You should also avoid or decrease intake of foods that can increase magnesium excretion, such as refined carbohydrates (white bread, white rice, etc.). Eating a diet that is high in fats, proteins, and phosphorus can also decrease your body's magnesium absorption.

Other foods that rob your body of magnesium include:

- Caffeine
- Sugar
- Alcohol
- Soft drinks
- Tea
- Rhubarb
- Spinach
- Cocoa

Eat Foods Rich in Vitamin D

Most people drink milk that's been fortified with vitamin D. However, vitamin D milk and dairy foods can cause magnesium absorption to decrease. Without enough magnesium, the active form of vitamin D in the blood is reduced.

Vitamin D is a fat-soluble vitamin that is actually manufactured in our skin as it comes in contact with the sun's ultraviolet rays. It is found mainly in meat products—especially in fish liver oils. Good dietary sources of vitamin D include egg yolks, butter, cod liver oil, salmon, mackerel, herring, and other meats. Artificial fats, such as olestra, may prevent vitamin D from being absorbed. Also fat-blockers such as chitosan or the fat-blocking weight-loss drug orlistat (Xenical or Alli) may also decrease absorption of vitamin D.

Vitamin D is required for your body to absorb calcium and phosphorus and to maintain normal levels of calcium and phosphorous in your bloodstream. Vitamin D also helps in bone mineralization. Without adequate vitamin D, bones may become brittle and thin. Vitamin D is very important for the transport of calcium from the intestines into the blood. It also decreases the excretion of calcium from the kidneys and helps the bones mineralize.

For the past forty-plus years most doctors have been recommending that two to three large glasses of milk be consumed every day, which provides between 600 and 900 milligrams of calcium. However, drinking milk may not be the best way for your body to get necessary vitamin D. Sunlight and eating foods with vitamin D are better sources of vitamin D because they do not inhibit magnesium absorption as does drinking milk.

PREVENT OSTEOPOROSIS WITH HEALTHY EATING

- Do not eat a lot of meats.
- Chocolate, spinach, rhubarb, cashews, asparagus, beet greens, and chard (high in oxalic acid) will inhibit the absorption of calcium; therefore, it is best to not take calcium supplements at the same time.
- Whole grains and fiber can also bind calcium. Therefore, it is best not to take calcium supplements at the same time.
- Decrease intake of alcohol, coffee, tea, colas, and other caffeinated beverages.
- Decrease salt intake.

Our skin makes vitamin D when we are exposed to UVB radiation from the sun. Usually the daily requirement of vitamin D can be obtained from being in the sunlight for approximately ten to fifteen minutes at midday wearing shorts and a T-shirt. Dark-skinned individuals require approximately five times more sun exposure in order to get the same amount of vitamin D as a fair-skinned person. Because they get less exposure to sunshine, people living in northern states are more likely to be deficient in vitamin D.

Very few foods contain any significant amounts of vitamin D naturally.

The Importance of Exercise

Exercise can help not only prevent osteoporosis, but it can also help treat it by providing strength to your bones and muscles. Exercise slows mineral loss, helps you maintain good posture, and improves your overall fitness, which reduces the risk of falls.

Weight-bearing exercises and strengthening exercises are the most important forms of exercise in treating osteoporosis. However, using weights or doing calisthenics to build muscles will also help to build bones. Realize the stronger your muscles are, generally the stronger your bones are.

Human bones are constantly being remodeled and reformed, but this remodeling happens in response to the demands and stresses that are placed on the bone by exercise. Weight-bearing exercises will actually stimulate the growth of new bone cells. The bones, however, must be stressed in order to grow. Weight-bearing exercise will not only stop bone loss but will also increase the mass of bone.

A sedentary lifestyle leads eventually to death for your bones. Many women develop osteoporosis despite having had adequate amounts of calcium in their diets. Why?

They don't stress their bones adequately through exercise. As a result, they lose significant amounts of bone.

Weight-bearing exercises such as dancing, walking, running, stair climbing, team sports, and yard work are often recommended in fighting osteoporosis. They are beneficial because they will stress (and thereby strengthen) the leg bones and hip bones. However, these activities are not as beneficial in preventing osteoporosis in the upper body—the spine, arms, and so forth.

The only exercises that prevent osteoporosis in the entire skeleton are weight-bearing exercises such as weight lifting and calisthenics. Weight-bearing exercises force you to work against gravity. Bicycling and swimming, while excellent for building muscle and improving the health of your cardiovascular system, do much less to build bone.

While a gym and trainer might be beyond your budget, a low-cost option is to purchase dumbbells and a DVD that can guide you to create a basic weight lifting program right in your own home. Performing calisthenics such as push-ups, or even lifting a five-pound bag of sugar, a can of paint, or a gallon of bottled water over your head will go a long way in improving your overall bone health.

You can try to do every one of these recommendations and still miss out on healthy bones if you do not also pay attention to your psychological and spiritual needs. The wisdom of Scripture explains:

> A merry heart does good like a medicine, but a broken spirit dries the bones.
> —PROVERBS 17:22

A happy women is much more likely to have strong bones than one who is depressed or angry. Are you taking your "merry heart" bone medicine daily?

Chapter 10

WEIGHT MANAGEMENT

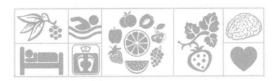

WEIGHT LOSS HAS become a national obsession in America. Women of every age are constantly trying to lose weight through diets, exercise, herbal remedies, behavior modification, and more. It is unfortunate that this obsession is often triggered by concerns about appearance instead of health. Sadly, women often turn to fashion rather than health when it comes to determining their ideal weight.

If you think you need to start dieting, you are not alone. Just look at the number of fad diets out there. The age-old wisdom of "eat less and exercise more" hasn't been popular enough to launch any diet book onto the best-seller list. What does sell, however, is any book that promises some new "miracle" or "breakthrough" method for easy weight loss. While there may be one or two good points about each of the new, popular fad diets on the market today, by and large, they don't produce long-term results. They may even prove to be risky to your health rather than beneficial.

So Much Food

It is important that you understand that all foods do not have the same effect on the body. Carbohydrates, found in many foods, but particularly abundant in grains and rice, metabolize into sugar at different rates. Those that waste no time, such as a big chocolate chip cookie, are called high-glycemic carbohydrates. Those that take their time, such as vegetables, are categorized as low-glycemic carbohydrates. Why does it matter?

Sugar in the bloodstream sends a signal to the pancreas to release the hormone insulin. When there is a lot of sugar, insulin levels become very high. Insulin has a big job to do and can choose to do it in several ways; the bottom line is that it must reduce the sugar (glucose) in the bloodstream. Some glucose is used by the cells as fuel for energy production, but insulin also sees to it that any excess glucose is stored as a fat cell for future use. After a large meal or a high-glycemic snack, insulin becomes particularly plentiful and efficient and quickly reduces blood sugar—so much, in fact, that it leaves you in short supply.

Sensing you now don't have enough sugar to function properly (you are light-headed and hungry), your body goes into alarm mode telling you to search for something to eat, preferably something you instinctively know will give you a fast boost—something sweet. You down a doughnut, insulin again pours into your system, and this feast or famine cycle is repeated again and again. Every insulin cycle squirrels away a few more fat cells in preparation for the day you can't find a snack. The result for all but a lucky 25 percent of the population, whose carbohydrate intake has little effect on their metabolism, is weight gain, especially for another 25 percent who appear very sensitive to weight gain after eating carbohydrates.

The more processed the food, the more quickly it is digested—a doughnut versus a slice of Irish brown bread, for example. To slow things down, select fruit over fruit juices or soft drinks. Eat pasta slightly under cooked—like the Italians. Add vinegar or lemon juice to carbohydrate foods; the acid slows their rate of absorption about 30 percent. Opt for sourdough or grainy bread—bagels can't wait to become sugar. Choose slow-cooked oatmeal and "all bran" over processed cereals.

> Watch your portion size. Make a fist, which is the size of the amount of protein you should eat at each meal. Two fists indicate the amount of fruit, vegetables, and healthy grains eaten at each meal. One thumb is the amount of healthy fat that should be eaten at each meal (such as olive oil or flaxseed oil).

Some people crave carbohydrates because of their ability to improve mood. Carbohydrates increase the production of serotonin. That piece of chocolate cake works as a natural tranquilizer or antidepressant, but with the side effect of extra fat. The urge to grab a "goodie" to allay fear, anxiety, or sadness isn't just lack of will power; it has biological roots.

Women need to know that falling levels of estrogen lower insulin secretion and decrease insulin sensitivity, a partial explanation for why you tend to gain weight at midlife. Progesterone increases insulin secretion and insulin resistance, offering a partial explanation for carbohydrate cravings before a monthly period. To avoid the carbohydrate roller coaster, blood sugar levels must be maintained throughout the day. You can do this by eating frequent smaller meals and being careful in your selection of carbohydrates, which must be balanced by proper portions of protein and fat to slow absorption and help you feel full.

Risks of Being Overweight

Everyone knows that it's not good to be overweight. But it's not just a matter of how you look. Did you know that being just ten to twenty pounds overweight increases your risk of premature death? Those excess pounds increase your risk of heart disease, diabetes, cancer, asthma, and other illnesses. In fact, every two-pound increase in weight increases the risk of arthritis by at least 9 percent, and a woman who gains more than twenty pounds after age eighteen doubles her risk of postmenopausal breast cancer. A weight gain of just eleven pounds will double the risk of acquiring type 2 diabetes.

Your body mass index (BMI) is a useful indicator for determining whether you are at increased risk for health problems associated with being overweight or obese. Generally the higher your BMI (your height to weight ratio) the higher your health risk. (See chapter 14 to find out how to calculate your BMI.[1])

Your health risk can also be assessed by figuring your waist/hip ratio. To do so, simply measure around the fullest part of your buttocks. Then measure your waist at the narrowest part of your torso. Now divide your waist measurement by your hip measurement. A healthy ratio is less than 0.8. The ideal ratio is 0.74. If your ratio is greater than 0.85, your health is at risk.

To find out your percentage of body fat, you may purchase a scale that measures your weight and body fat percentage (they are fairly accurate), or you can have it measured at a health club or by your physician. A body fat percentage between 20 and 28 is considered healthy for women in their premenopausal or menopausal years, while 12 to 23 percent is ideal for younger women.

Older and Heavier

Americans aged sixty to seventy-four years old are gaining weight faster than any other age group. While it is true that your risk of dying sooner is only slightly higher if you are obese compared to your same-age slim friend, that is only part of the story. The rest of the story is quality of life. The closer you are to your ideal weight, the greater your energy, mobility, and likelihood of independence will be as you age.

Much of what is considered "aging" is loss of muscle. Muscle loss occurs naturally, and muscle is harder to maintain as we get older. As we become weaker and less active, loss escalates. You gain weight because muscle burns more calories than fat, and with the loss of muscle, your fat-burning machine is missing. Therefore, building and maintaining muscle is crucial to maintaining and losing weight.

Quick weight loss can result in breaking down muscle rather than fat. You may look trim, but the ratio of muscle to body fat has shifted, and keeping weight off becomes increasingly difficult. Muscles are also a source of protein; loss of protein in muscles means loss of function elsewhere. If you happen to become ill, you have fewer muscle cells for the manufacture of antibodies, wound healing, and white blood cell production.

Can You Speed Up Your Metabolism?

The speed at which our metabolism functions is influenced by many factors: age, gender, heredity, and proportion of lean body mass. The older we get, the slower our metabolism functions. After age forty, the metabolism slows 5 percent per decade. Metabolism establishes the rate at which we burn calories and how efficiently the body uses the fuel it is fed through food. Hormones and enzymes are what convert food into fuel, and there are ways to supplement the hormones and enzymes you need to boost your sluggish metabolism.

An amino acid manufactured in your liver, acetyl L-carnitine (ALC) helps facilitate fat metabolism, increases energy production in muscle cells, promotes fat loss, and increases circulation in the brain. In other words, the body uses ALC to turn fat into energy. Acetyl L-carnitine and carnitine are widely available in animal foods and dairy products, but plant-based foods have very small amounts. It can be taken as a pill, but carnitine alone is not able to cross the blood-brain barrier as well as its activated form, acetyl L-carnitine.

Your thyroid gland is your body's metabolic pacemaker. When your thyroid fails to produce enough thyroid hormone, your body's metabolism slows down, causing the following symptoms (known as hypothyroidism): fatigue, depression, weakness, weight gain, high cholesterol levels, low body temperature, and hair loss. It is estimated that one in four American women can attribute their weight gain to low or borderline low thyroid hormones. Women with healthy thyroid function burn calories more efficiently. When your thyroid hormone levels are restored, your energy level, weight, temperature, muscle strength, cholesterol, emotional health, and more will improve.

Thyroid conditions can be effectively treated with medication. It may take a few weeks or months to find just the right dose. The natural supplement L-tyrosine plays a crucial role in supporting the thyroid gland. Tyrosine boosts your metabolism as well as acting as the precursor for dopamine, norepinephrine, and epinephrine, which are nervous system chemicals that affect metabolism, mental alertness, and energy levels. Tyrosine can be taken in supplement form with a meal that contains protein. If your doctor finds that you are suffering from hypothyroidism, you may take L-tyrosine with your thyroid medication. Make sure to keep your thyroid monitored with periodic blood tests. You may be able to reduce or eliminate the need for the medication.

Weight-Related Health Concerns

The National Institutes of Health and the US Surgeon General declare "the top ten causes of death due to disease are attributable to health risks associated with excess body fat." The NIH states, "Obesity is a leading cause of heart disease, hypertension, stroke, diabetes and even cancer."[2]

Age has something to do with it. After age thirty the rate at which we break down our food and the efficiency with which we utilize or store it begin to slow down, about 1 percent a year. As a result of a lower metabolism and the fact that we tend to begin slowdown in our exercise routines, weight stealthily increases unless the simple decision is made to eat less and exercise more.

It's a fact of life: at about fifty everything starts to slow down: stamina, hair growth, thinking, and metabolism. Other midlife menaces join the party: heartburn, gastroesophageal reflux disease (GERD), acid reflux, indigestion, bloating, gas, constipation, fatigue. When digestion is not optimal, energy is reduced and constipation, bloating, gas, reflux, allergic reactions, and nausea can be constant companions.

Weight gain at midlife can set the stage for some of the most serious health threats of our time, including cancer, heart disease, and diabetes. When you add stress, which can result in excess cortisol production, you may gain twenty or so midlife pounds that seem impossible to lose.

The Cortisol-Obesity Connection

Studies suggest a link between central obesity, marked by abdominal fat and a high waist-to-hip ratio, to elevated cortisol levels. Exercise, stress-management techniques such as relaxation and medication, and nutritional supplements can help you manage stress and lower cortisol to promote optimal health and longevity. The following are scientifically supported techniques that can help support a healthy response to stress.

Behavioral techniques to lower stress and manage high cortisol levels:

- Exercise 30–45 minutes of both anaerobic (resistance training) and aerobic (jogging, cycling) every other day.
- Meditation relaxation: 15–30 minutes daily

Supplements to reduce high cortisol levels secondary to stress:

- Vitamin C: 1,000–3,000 milligrams a day
- Fish oil (omega-3 fatty acids): 1–4 milligrams a day
- Phosphatidylserine: 300–800 milligrams a day

- Rhodiola rosea: 100–200 milligrams a day, standardized extract
- Ginseng: 100–300 milligrams a day, standardized extract
- Ginkgo biloba: 100–200 milligrams a day, standardized extract
- DHEA: 25–50 milligrams a day (any hormone supplementation should be monitored by your physician)[3]

Gradual weight loss is more permanent than quick weight loss. The results are more likely to be permanent if the weight loss is a daily gradual process of lifestyle and dietary changes.

American Women and Weight Management

Weight control is all-important to a woman's health and happiness, but a woman's weight issues cannot be addressed successfully until she has accepted her body unconditionally. Women need to regain the body acceptance and self-esteem that they lose as they enter adolescence. Here are some ideas toward developing better weight control:

- Try to befriend your body just as it is, and list five things you like about your body right now. Remind yourself of those items the next time you are feeling self-critical.
- Perfect your posture; stand tall, and walk with grace. Dress to play up your best features.
- Continue to take charge of your health. Get in the habit of scanning your body once a day, paying attention to areas in which you feel pain or tension. Long before an illness develops, your body often sends you warning signals. Paying attention to them will help you to maintain a high energy level as well as prevent a bigger health crisis. Keep up with medical screening tests—blood pressure, breast, skin, and cholesterol checks; Pap smears; and dental checkups.
- Do not deprive yourself. Make sure you eat plenty of fruits, vegetables, and whole grains for lifetime protection from all sorts of chronic diseases, as well as to help keep your weight in balance. When you crave chocolate, indulge! Just don't overdo it!
- Everyone gets overstressed from time to time, whether from family obligations, work, or just too much to do. When your body and soul become depleted, you need rest, along with emotional and spiritual sustenance to get back on an even keel. Make time to catch up on your sleep. Spend

quality time with a good friend. Enjoy a romantic dinner. Escape for a long weekend alone or spend a day gardening—whatever works for you.

The following dietary guidelines are designed to help you choose the foods that can most help you achieve balance in your weight. First, it is important to consume high-fiber foods. Fiber improves the excretion of fat, improves glucose tolerance, and gives you a feeling of fullness and satisfaction. Emphasize the following foods: brown rice, tuna, chicken, white fish, fresh fruits and vegetables, high-protein lean foods, lentils, beans, whole-grain bread, and turkey. Add healthy fats to your diet, such as olive oil, safflower oil, and flax oil. Whey protein shakes can help to keep blood sugar stabilized and fat-burning. Avoid sugars and snack foods that contain salt and fat, such as potato chips, ice cream, candy, cookies, cake, breakfast cereals that are high in sugar, and soda. Do not choose high-fat cheeses, sour cream, whole milk, butter, mayonnaise, fried foods, peanut butter (unless it is natural), or rich salad dressings. Do not drink alcoholic beverages at all—they are high in calories and worsen any number of health problems.

Eat several small meals daily instead of skipping meals and eating one big meal daily. You want to give your body even burning fuel throughout the day. Otherwise your body will store fat for "survival" instead of burning it.

Soup is a great way to get high-nutrient, high-fiber foods into your meals. Eating homemade, nutritious soup that is low in salt will not only nourish you but will also flush waste from your body. A serving of low-calorie, high-fiber soup such as vegetable soup or minestrone has only around 75 to 125 calories.

VERY VEGGIE SLIMMING SOUP

2 Tbsp. olive oil	2 large carrots, sliced
1 large onion, chopped	1 zucchini, chopped
2 green and/or red bell peppers, chopped	1 yellow squash, chopped
4 garlic cloves, minced	1 can (14½ oz.) low-sodium stewed tomatoes
½ tsp. ground cumin	1 bottle (46 oz.) vegetable juice
½ small head cabbage, sliced	½ tsp. ground black pepper

Warm oil in a large saucepan over medium heat. Add onion and bell peppers. Cook five minutes or until tender. Add garlic and cumin. Cook one minute. Add cabbage, carrots, zucchini, squash, tomatoes (with juice), vegetable juice, black pepper, and red pepper flakes. Heat to boiling. Reduce heat to low, cover, and simmer one hour.

New fad diets come along every few years, such as the Atkins diet, the Ornish diet, the South Beach diet, the Zone diet, the sugar busters diet, the blood type diet, the Paleolithic diet, and…well, you get the idea. When it comes right down to it, most of the new fad diets are actually harmful to a person's health. They tend to run to one extreme or the other, advocating excessive amounts of cholesterol, saturated fat, or animal protein. They also tend to be lacking in many key nutrients necessary to counter disease. Other potential dangerous effects that have been noted include:

- Mild dehydration
- Headaches
- Nausea
- Sleep problems
- Fatigue
- Increased risk of osteoporosis
- Inability to maintain weight loss
- High blood pressure

Whole Foods or "Live Foods"

A whole-food live diet promotes health by decreasing fats and sugar intake while increasing fiber and nutrient intake. This means more satisfaction and less overeating. Whole-food diets are low in fat and cholesterol but high in essential nutrients—unlike foods many Americans normally eat that rob the body rather than nourish it; for example, refined sugars, commercial colas, refined-grain flours and pastas, processed fats, hydrogenated fats such as margarine, and deep-fried foods.

A whole-food diet is generously filled with live foods in their whole state. This is the way we were intended to eat—different colored vegetables and fruits; grains; raw seeds, nuts and their butters; beans; fermented dairy products such as yogurt and kefir; fish; poultry; and bean products such as tofu. A whole-foods diet should be lower in cheeses and fats as well as animal meats. By eating a whole-food diet, you will be consuming a diet that is high in foods as whole as possible with the least amount of processed, adulterated, fried, or sweetened additives.

Did you know that many of the foods at your local grocery store have been picked or slaughtered weeks or even *months* before they reach your store? They are often artificially preserved or treated with nitrogen to help deter spoilage. The longer it takes for foods to get to your table means diminished nutrition for you and your family. What can you do? Start shopping at farmer's markets whenever possible. Make it a point to:

- Eat more high-protein plant foods—nuts, grains, seeds, and legumes.
- Choose free-range, hormone-free, additive-free meats.

- Have rhythm to your diet. Eating regularly provides your body with a consistent intake of nutrient-dense foods and will therefore prevent you from overeating and reaching for "dead," over processed, sugar-laden foods.

- Eat fresh and in season.

Through the combination of eating the right foods, burning calories through physical exercise, and supplementing the diet with the proper nutrients, it is possible to lose the weight and keep it off. And not only can you do it without any detrimental effects to your body, but your health also will actually improve as a result of the changes that you make.

Food winners

As scientists continue to study the chemistry of the human body, several common groups of foods have been proven to increase metabolism and block the fatty acid uptake in the body's cells, thus causing a person to lose weight.

- Oatmeal. The fiber found in common oatmeal has an incredible impact on the insulin levels in the bloodstream. When you eat sugary foods, the insulin converts those carbohydrates into fat storage and slows down your metabolism. But the fiber present in oatmeal blunts that insulin response. Have a bowl of oatmeal, or another type of oat bran cereal that is high in fiber, for breakfast. Fiber supplements such as apple pulp concentrate, citrus pectin and glucomannan, from the konjac plant, can also have the same effect.

- Green tea. Certain chemicals within the green teas commonly found in Asian countries have been shown to increase the body's metabolic rate and increase the breakdown and elimination of fat. The polyphenols present in the tea have a thermogenic effect on the body; that is, it causes the body to begin to burn its fat reservoirs. The amount of caffeine that is present in green tea, unlike the amount found in coffee, doesn't cause the jitters, but it does increase metabolism and allows the body to burn more calories while resting.

- Protein. Diets that restrict protein intake are missing one important fact: protein requires more calories to digest in the body than do carbohydrates or fats. To a certain extent, shifting to a higher protein diet will burn more calories and cause you to lose more weight. It is important not to go to an extreme with this, however, because too much protein can be harmful to the kidneys. It is also better to obtain protein in your diet from low-fat sources such as poultry and fish rather than from red meats.

• Fish. The omega-3 fatty acids present in fish such as salmon, trout, mackerel, cod, and sardines have consistently been shown to increase body metabolism.

Increased body metabolism is important because it increases the rate at which the body can burn fat while at rest. In other words, you can be "working off" those calories just by sitting in your chair! In fact, 65 to 70 percent of the total calories that you burn are burned while at rest, just to keep the heart beating, your intestines working, your food being digested in your system and other "automatic" processes. However, if you hope to lose weight and maintain good health, burning metabolic calories alone is not enough. Physical activity should be an important factor in any weight-loss plan.

The Importance of Physical Activity

Studies have shown that lifting weights two or three times per week increases strength by building muscle mass and bone density. For example, a twelve-month study conducted at Tufts University demonstrated 1 percent gains in hip and spine density, 75 percent increases in strength, and 13 percent increases in dynamic balance with just two days per week of progressive strength training. The control group had losses in both strength and balance.[4] The good news, especially for women, is that strength training can help to prevent long-term medical problems such as osteoporosis. Strength training uses resistance methods such as free weights, weight machines, and resistance bands to build muscles and strength.

You can combine strength training with your aerobic activity by using handheld weights or ankle weights when you walk. If you have bone or joint problems, you may do leg lifts, wall push-ups, and traditional push-ups.

Overcoming Midlife Weight Gain

The most beautiful season of the year is autumn. But too many women think of the autumn season of their lives as a time of loss: losing one's youth, one's figure, one's energy and stamina. One way to embrace this time of life is to make it all it can be through determined effort. Your body will respond to your control as you master it. Your body needs to be maintained in health through weight loss and exercise. Obesity is a major cause of estrogen dominance, which leads to premenopausal symptoms. As you recall, fatty tissue will cause an increased production of estrogen.

TEN QUICK STRENGTH-TRAINING TIPS

1. Remember to warm up. Warming up gives the body a chance to deliver plenty of nutrient-rich blood to areas about to be exercised to actually warm the muscles and lubricate the joints.

2. Stretching increases or maintains muscle flexibility.

3. During the first week of starting an exercise program keep it light. Work on technique and good body mechanics, and slowly work up to heavier weights.

4. Quick tips to maintain good body mechanics: go through the complete range of motion, move slowly and with control, breathe, and maintain a neutral spine. Never sacrifice form just to add more weight or repetitions.

5. The intensity of your workout depends on a number of factors, including the number of sets and repetitions, the overall weight lifted, and the rest between sets. You can vary the intensity of your workout to fit your activity level and goals.

6. Listen to your body. Heart rate is not a good way to determine your intensity when lifting weights; it is important to listen to your body based on an overall sense or feeling of exertion.

7. The minimum amount of strength training recommended by the American College of Sports Medicine is eight to twelve repetitions of eight to ten exercises, at a moderate intensity, two days a week. You will get more overall gains with more days per week, sets, and resistance, but the progression is one in which you must listen to your body.

8. Strength-training sessions are recommended to last one hour or less.

9. As a general rule each muscle that you train should be rested one to two days before being exercised further in order for the fatigued muscles to rebuild.

10. "No pain, no gain." This statement is not only false, but it can also be dangerous. Your body will adapt to strength training and will reduce in body soreness each time you work out.[5]

Try taking a twenty- to thirty-minute brisk walk every other day. Or find another exercise that you enjoy and can do at least three to four times a week. Regular exercise can make all the difference during this season of your life. It helps keep your metabolism high, which prevents weight gain, and it reduces the effects and intensity of hot flashes.

Most people feel calm and have a sense of well-being after they exercise. You can actually walk off your anxieties. People who exercise feel better about themselves, look better, feel more energetic, and are more productive at work.

What Would You Like to Weigh?

Suppose you could wake up tomorrow morning with the body weight that is perfect for you. What would that be? You may have given up on enjoying your ideal body weight a long time ago. You shouldn't have. Now is the best time for you to enjoy your life! So set a goal.

Find your height and frame size on the chart below and make note of your goal weight.

My goal weight is ___ pounds.
My actual weight is ___ pounds.
I need to lose ___ pounds.

HEIGHT AND WEIGHT TABLE FOR WOMEN			
Height	Small Frame	Medium Frame	Large Frame
4'10"	102–111 lbs.	109–121 lbs.	118–131 lbs.
4'11"	103–113 lbs.	111–123 lbs.	120–134 lbs.
5'0"	104–115 lbs.	113–126 lbs.	122–137 lbs.
5'1"	106–118 lbs.	115–129 lbs.	125–140 lbs.
5'2"	108–121 lbs.	118–132 lbs.	128–143 lbs.
5'3"	111–124 lbs.	121–135 lbs.	131–147 lbs.
5'4"	114–127 lbs.	124–138 lbs.	134–151 lbs.
5'5"	117–130 lbs.	127–141 lbs.	137–155 lbs.
5'6"	120–133 lbs.	130–144 lbs.	140–159 lbs.
5'7"	123–136 lbs.	133–147 lbs.	143–163 lbs.
5'8"	126–139 lbs.	136–150 lbs.	146–167 lbs.
5'9"	129–142 lbs.	139–153 lbs.	149–170 lbs.
5'10"	132–145 lbs.	142–156 lbs.	152–173 lbs.
5'11"	135–148 lbs.	145–159 lbs.	155–176 lbs.
6'0"	138–151 lbs.	148–162 lbs.	158–179 lbs.

Lifestyle Changes to Support Weight Loss

It will be important for you to make the following lifestyle changes to be successful in your weight-loss program:

- Avoid fad diets, which do not work and give only temporary results.

- Eat slowly and chew your food properly. Take time to taste your food.

- Do not eat when you are upset, lonely, or depressed.

- Chewing gum can stimulate your appetite, so you should leave it alone while trying to lose weight.

- Drink plenty of water.

- Stay regular. Do not become constipated.

- Begin a walking program (after dinner is best).

SIMPLE RULES FOR WEIGHT AND HEALTH MANAGEMENT

- Graze on salads and veggies often throughout the day.
- Eat a fairly large breakfast.
- Eat smaller midmorning, midafternoon, and evening snacks.
- Avoid all simple sugar foods such as candies, cookies, cakes, pies and doughnuts. If you must have sugar, use either Stevia or Sweet Balance (found in health food stores).
- Drink two quarts of water a day.
- Avoid alcohol.
- Avoid all fried foods and decrease intake of animal fats (whole milk, cheese, fatty cuts of meat, bacon, sausage, ham, etc.).
- Avoid, or decrease dramatically, starches. Starches include all breads, crackers, bagels, potatoes, pasta, rice, and corn.
- Eat high-fiber foods.
- Eat fresh fruits; steamed, stir-fried, or raw vegetables; lean meats; salads (preferably with extra-virgin olive oil and vinegar); nuts (almonds, organic peanuts), and seeds.
- Do not eat past 7:00 p.m.

The key thing to remember about weight loss is balance. Make sure each meal and snack contain carbohydrates to provide glucose for your brain, protein to provide amino acids needed to build and repair body protein and release glucagon (your fat-burning hormone), and fat to supply fatty acids needed for blood sugar control, appetite suppression, and hormone production.

....

Bless the LORD, O my soul, and forget not all His benefits....
Who satisfies your mouth with good things, so that your
youth is renewed like the eagle's. —Psalm 103:2, 5

....

Chapter 11

MEMORY AND MENTAL CLARITY

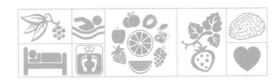

HAVE YOU EVER forgotten someone's name? Lost your car keys? All of us show signs of forgetfulness from time to time, especially as we get older, and it can be worrisome—where is the line drawn between simple forgetfulness and a symptom of a more dangerous, more frightening prospect—Alzheimer's disease or another neurological disorder?

The problem of neurological impairment—including Alzheimer's disease, dementia, and severe memory loss—is on the rise. Reports suggest that in the next twenty-five years, the incidence of Alzheimer's disease will triple. Already 50 percent of the population that attains the age of eighty-five shows the signs of early Alzheimer's. Almost everyone over the age of forty has some degree of age-related memory loss and this forgetfulness causes people to worry about losing their minds.

The key to determining whether or not the problem is serious is to determine whether or not it is *progressive.* To determine the cause of a possible problem, doctors use a standard memory test. They will state three words aloud to the patient—such as run, blue, table—and then tell the person that they will be asked to repeat those words two minutes later in the conversation. Whether or not the patient can complete this task successfully tells the doctor a great deal about the functioning of the memory centers of the patient's brain.

When the doctor states the words, they are stored as a memory in the entorhinal cortex of the brain, and then sent to the hippocampus, where longer-term memories are stored. Because Alzheimer's affects these areas of the brain first, it is possible to pinpoint potential early Alzheimer's patients if they fail the test.

Naturally some degree of forgetfulness can be caused by distraction or a lack of attention at the time the information is given. The distraction prevents the listener from incorporating what was heard and moving it into the memory centers of the brain. For that reason doctors will additionally ask the patient about memories from his or her childhood. If the patient cannot pull up these memories as well, it is a strong indication that something is causing a serious impairment in the brain. Most early Alzheimer's patients will be able to recall childhood memories, but the majority of them will not be able to repeat the list of words. The testers work backward to find out where the degree of forgetfulness begins, and then they determine the level of impairment from there.

ARE YOU EXPERIENCING MEMORY LOSS?

Take the following test to determine if you are experiencing memory loss.

- Do you often forget a common word that you use every day and substitute another one in its place?
- Do you go looking for something, only to forget what it was you were searching for?
- Do you forget the names of friends?
- Do you forget appointments?
- Do you forget the point you were trying to make while talking?
- Do you misplace keys?
- Do you find it increasingly difficult to learn new things?
- Do you find it difficult to add numbers in your head?
- Do you have difficulty concentrating?
- Do you depend upon caffeine to be mentally keen?
- Do you always feel fatigued?
- Do petty problems frustrate you?
- Do you frequently repeat yourself?
- Do you occasionally get lost while driving, even if you have driven there numerous times before?
- Does your family think that you are more forgetful now compared to before?

If you identified nine or more, you probably have age-associated memory impairment. If you relate to twelve or more, you may have early Alzheimer's disease.[1]

Other Symptoms of Serious Memory Impairment

Besides short-term memory loss, cognitive tests include problems with simple arithmetic. Alzheimer's patients have great difficulty performing calculations or simple arithmetic in their minds. These are not calculations such as finding a square root. These calculations are the simple addition and subtraction problems that we learned as children, such as two plus five equals seven.

Just because your old uncle Joe likes to retell his famous fishing story over and over about when he caught the biggest bass in the county, it doesn't mean that he is in the early stages of Alzheimer's. But if people repeat the same story over and over again because they can't remember that they just told it five minutes ago, it signals a problem. If a person asks the same question over and over again because they don't remember having asked it moments prior, some degree of short-term memory loss has developed. If a person has taken the same route home from work for ten years, but one day cannot remember which way to go, it is another warning sign.

> ## MEMORY LAPSES OF MENOPAUSE
>
> The brain's neurotransmitters are influenced by estrogen. Inability to re-member words and names of things can be a sign of estrogen in short sup-ply. Changes in memory and concentration are noted at menopause be-cause the hippocampus (learning and memory center) depends on estro-gen to interact with its many estrogen receptors.

Poor judgment is another telling symptom. This is not the poor judgment that a young person might have when he or she makes bad decisions because of immaturity. When people forget to bathe or begin to wear soiled clothing, they are exercising poor judgment because of their mental state. Another example is when an individual con-tinually forgets to turn off the oven or leaves the car running in the driveway because he or she forgot to turn the motor off.

Forgetting the names of strangers or one-time acquaintances does not usually signal a significant problem. However, a person has already developed a serious problem when he or she can't remember the name of an aunt or uncle or closest friend of thirty years—or even his or her own mother or child.

Any one of these symptoms alone may not be an indication of a serious problem, but if more than one symptom begins to manifest and if there are signs of progressive memory loss, it's time to consider getting some help for the problem.

Wanted: Brain Cells (Not Dead, but Alive)

More than sixty diseases are capable of causing dementia. However, Alzheimer's dis-ease is responsible for more dementia than all other causes combined. Alzheimer's disease causes major changes in a person's brain tissue. First, the brain cells develop abnormal fibers called neurofibrillary tangles. These tangles interfere with the function of the brain cells and eventually kill them. In addition, the brain cells accumulate senile plaques, which are dead cellular material that accumulate around a protein (amyloid).

Until not long ago the medical community has believed that once a neuron, a nerve cell, died—including the cells of the brain—it could never be regenerated or brought back to life. They believed the body could heal itself in every other tissue or organ, but once damage was done in the brain, it was irreversible. Therefore, common wisdom said that nothing could be done about memory loss. It was just a fact of growing old.

Then scientists began to learn that brain cells, or neurons, can and do regenerate under the proper conditions. Now PET and SPECT scans can map brain activity and measure both the destruction and growth of new brain cells. What these experts discovered was absolutely fascinating—and it completely changed the way we think about memory loss. Thanks to these marvelous advances, today we know that even damaged brains can grow new cells.[2]

GREEN TEA

Green tea contains antioxidants called polyphenols, which increase antioxidant activity in the blood up to 50 percent. Green tea is also rich in flavonoids, which can help prevent blood clots and may reduce the incidence of mini-strokes, which also cause memory loss. Many different kinds of flavonoids exist, including bioflavonoids, pine bark extract, and grape seed extract.

To a lesser extent, black tea, from which most of teas on the market are made, has similar antioxidant properties. In black tea, the tea leaves have been allowed to oxidize, which reduces the potency of the polyphenols. Drink two to three cups of green tea per day. But don't drink it in the evenings since it contains some caffeine, which may interfere with your ability to sleep.

Menopausal "Senior Moments"

The memory loss associated with aging is called age-associated memory impairment, but many seniors prefer to say they are simply having a "senior moment." But be careful not to confuse terms. Dementia, although once called senility, is memory impairment on a much greater scale.

And neither one may be your problem if you are menopausal. Just as with PMS, one of the symptoms of menopause can be a problem with mental clarity. Just when you think you're doing fine, you realize that you have a black shoe on your left foot and a navy one on your right. You may not trace it back to your week of short sleep (due to night sweats) or your regrettable junk food binge, but your body—and your mind—may be in survival mode. You and your hormones never saw it coming.

Work Out for Brain Health

Exercise can help prevent mental decline. Most of us know that physical exercise is good for our general health, but did you know that physical exercise is also good for your brain? If you think you're going to get smarter sitting in front of your computer or watching television, think again. Physical exercise has a protective effect on the brain and its mental processes, and it may even help prevent Alzheimer's disease. Based on exercise and health data from nearly five thousand men and women over sixty-five years of age, those who exercised were less likely to lose their mental abilities or develop dementia, including Alzheimer's. Furthermore, the more a person exercises, the greater the protective benefits for the brain, particularly in women. Inactive individuals in a recent study were twice as likely to develop Alzheimer's, compared to those with the highest levels of activity (those who exercised vigorously at least three times a week). But even light or moderate exercisers cut their risk significantly for Alzheimer's and mental decline.[3]

REGULAR PHYSICAL EXERCISE

- Increases brain cells
- Reduces the risk of Alzheimer's and dementia
- Improves sleep
- Strengthens memory
- Helps keep hormones in balance

If you have reached middle age or passed it and have never have exercised regularly, the good news is that it is not too late to start. Physical activity improves mental function by inducing the growth of capillaries, which are tiny blood vessels in the brain. Capillaries help nutrients reach neurons. This is very important because the aging process leads to a decrease in blood supply to the brain.

For decades, as mentioned above, it was considered a scientific fact that the brains of adult mammals had a fixed number of cells. This idea has been challenged by several studies that showed exercise nearly doubled the number of cells in the area of the brain involved with learning and memory, the hippocampus. This study was done on mice, but regeneration of the hippocampus has now been shown in adult birds and monkeys. One researcher speculated "intense exercise in a natural environment may be associated with a need for increased navigation skills." The hippocampus is thought to be the control center for the learning processes involved with navigating and understanding our surroundings.[4]

Physical exercise also leads to deep, recuperative sleep. It is during this deep sleep state that your brain gets the opportunity to consolidate memory and rebalance hormones and brain chemicals to get you ready for a new day. Exercise increases oxygen and glucose to the brain and helps to remove metabolic waste from the neurons of the brain. It helps increase the production of norepinephrine and dopamine, which are neurotransmitters that give you a sense of well-being.

Since the brain uses about 25 percent of your total blood oxygen, it's easy to see how exercising to increase the flow of oxygen to the brain is one of the easiest ways of improving your memory. Every step you take to improve your physical well-being will positively influence your brain health. Exercise is good not only for your body but also for your mind as well.

Free Radicals and Memory Loss

Because of the enormous amount of oxygen the brain requires, it also generates more free radicals than any other tissue in the body. Free radicals are a kind of molecular shrapnel.

Antioxidants stabilize free radicals before they can damage your body. But the brain appears to have a somewhat deficient natural supply of these defense weapons compared to the rest of the body. The brain forms large amounts of free radicals because the brain never stops working. Brain cells need a constant supply of both blood and oxygen. Therefore, significant amounts of free radicals are produced continually.

To understand free radicals, consider the process of oxidation. When you burn wood in a fireplace, smoke is a by-product. Likewise, when you metabolize food into energy, oxygen oxidizes (or burns) the food to produce energy. This process does not create smoke, but it does produce dangerous by-products known as free radicals. These are molecules with unpaired electrons that cause damage to other cells.

Free radicals can create cellular havoc in your brain, damaging many of the brain's functions.

Another culprit is called AGEs, or advanced glycosylation end products. AGEs are produced when the sugar (or glucose) in your blood reacts with proteins that are also in your blood. This reaction creates a protein substance that builds up in your cells in much the same way that plaque builds up on your teeth after a day of not brushing. This buildup is called AGEs.

SUPPLEMENTAL ANTIOXIDANTS

These antioxidants join together to form an impenetrable shield against free-radical attacks. When one antioxidant fails to neutralize a free-radical hit, another launches to back it up.

- Vitamin E
- Vitamin C
- Lipoic acid
- Glutathione
- Coenzyme Q_{10}

The higher the sugar levels in your diet, the more AGEs are created in your bloodstream. If you get enough of this sugar/protein buildup, you will actually age faster! It also creates brain-damaging free radicals that increase memory loss.

Antioxidants help defend the brain from free-radical damage. Many antioxidants are found naturally in fruits and vegetables. Those with the deepest color usually contain the highest amounts of antioxidants. Listed below are some fruits and vegetables in which you can find the highest level of antioxidants:

- Prunes
- Strawberries
- Garlic
- Spinach
- Cranberries
- Raspberries

Eating these fruits and vegetables will help save your brain from free-radical destruction. Some other powerful sources include grape juice, which has four times the antioxidant capacity of other juices, including grapefruit juice, tomato juice, and orange juice. However, it also contains sugar, so drinking too much can be detrimental. Black tea and green tea are very high in antioxidant potency. However, instant teas, herbal teas, and bottled teas have little or no antioxidant activity. Red wine is also full of antioxidants, but teas and red grape juice can give you as much protection as red wine, without the alcohol.

What If It Has Already Started?

Preventing further decline in memory is much easier than reversing it, and to reverse it, we need to understand what causes memory loss to occur as we age.

If you do nothing to halt or reverse the process, approximately 20 percent of all your brain cells will die over the course of your lifetime. Just as bone mass and muscle mass tend to shrink with age, this cell loss causes the brain mass to shrink as well. Between the ages of twenty and seventy, about 10 percent of brain mass will be lost.

THE FOLLOWING ACTIVITIES WILL EXERCISE YOUR BRAIN:

- Reading
- Playing chess, checkers, or board games
- Playing word games such as Scrabble
- Writing
- Getting involved in hobbies
- Conversing with your spouse or friends
- Studying a topic
- Listening to teaching

How Your Brain Works

Your thoughts are transmitted through your brain by cells called neurons. If you were able to get inside your brain, you would see that your brain cells look like an oak tree with thousands of branches, both large and very small. These brain cell branches are called dendrites. Dendrites branch out and connect with other brain cells. The more dendrites your brain has, the better your memory will be. And we now know that the brain is able to grow new dendrites, thus forming new thought pathways. This is why an individual who has suffered a stroke and has been paralyzed on one side can learn how to walk again. Even though the stroke killed brain cells, resulting in paralysis, new dendrite branches that were created by the brain went around the dead cells and restored the ability to walk.

Thinking and studying help to form new dendritic connections. That is why it is so critically important to keep mentally active; it is the only way to keep forming new dendritic connections.

Each brain cell or neuron is able to communicate with hundreds of thousands of other nerve cells at lightning speeds through *synapses,* the spaces that exist between the neurons or nerve cells. The synapses form a kind of electrical train where messages come in and go out along the nerve cells. Not only do brain cells grow new dendrites and receptors, but they also grow new synapses. We can create more message synapses, dendrites, and receptors through intentional activities such as obtaining proper and/or remedial nutrition, lowering stress, and doing physical and mental exercises. When our nerve cells have more synapses and dendrites with which to transmit brain messages, then we have quicker, more accurately functioning brains. Memory and other mental functioning can improve by increasing the connections among our brain cells.

The Necessity of Neurotransmitters

Neurons, the powerful cells that give us the ability to think and feel, transfer information to each other by using chemicals called neurotransmitters. Neurotransmitters are stored in vesicles (like little bags) inside the nerve cells and are released as needed. Different neurotransmitters have specific functions. They are released across the synapses and unite to receiver cells (receptor sites) on other nerve cells. In essence neurotransmitters convey a person's intelligence, memory, and mood.

Approximately fifty different varieties of these incredible chemicals have been identified in the brain. Some of the most important neurotransmitters include acetylcholine, norepinephrine, dopamine, serotonin, and GABA, some of which may sound familiar to the average person. Let's take a closer look at these brain chemicals.

Acetylcholine. The most important neurotransmitter for memory and thought is acetylcholine. If you have been experiencing difficulty concentrating, it may well be because your body lacks acetylcholine. Acetylcholine is made from choline, which is found in egg yolks. Your brain has more of this neurotransmitter than any other type. The brain of an Alzheimer's patient is also extremely deficient in this most important neurotransmitter.

Norepinephrine. Norepinephrine helps to transfer short-term memories to long-term storage. Norepinephrine also helps to elevate your mood. Your body is able to make its own norepinephrine from two important amino acids, L-tyrosine and L-phenylalanine.

Serotonin. Serotonin gives you a feeling of well-being and helps you sleep. You can increase the amount of serotonin in your body by eating tryptophan, which is an amino acid found in turkey, milk, cheese, legumes, cashews, dates, figs, bananas, and spinach.

Dopamine. Dopamine affects your memory, mood, and sex drive. People who have Parkinson's disease have very low dopamine levels. Dopamine helps the body to move freely (rather than rigidly as the bodies of Parkinson's patients tend to do).

GABA. GABA is a calming neurotransmitter and is critically important for sleep and relaxation. Without GABA, our minds would be overstimulated, and we would eventually become exhausted.

Which type of neurotransmitters that your neurons make and release is actually dependent upon what you eat? The brain is actually made up of fat. Believe it or not, it is the body's fattiest organ. About 60 percent of your brain is made from fatty substances called lipids. This makes it important to eat the proper kinds of fat to nourish the cells of your brain.

Diet for a Healthy Brain

Every brain cell is covered by a cell membrane composed of two layers of fats called phospholipids. Your brain cell membranes must be flexible and pliable to communicate easily and accurately with other cells in the brain. When you eat bad fats, such as saturated and hydrogenated fats, the brain cell membranes may become stiff and rigid.

Brain-enhancing fats

Foods containing omega-3 fats are brain enhancers. So for a keen mind load up your plate often with omega-3 choices such as the following:

- Fish oils
- Herring
- Salmon
- Tuna
- Mackerel
- Flaxseed oil
- Sardines

Omega-3s are the most fluid fats and thus help to keep brain cell membranes soft and pliable. If only 50 percent of your receptor sites are soft and pliable, then you may be getting only 50 percent of the messages your neurotransmitters are sending. This may be the reason why so many people lack razor-sharp minds—perhaps only half of their brain messages are able to get through.

One form of fish's omega-3 fatty acid is called DHA. It has been discovered that the more DHA a food contains, the higher the level of serotonin. Serotonin is a neurotransmitter that actually causes you to feel a greater sense of well-being. Prozac is also able to raise the serotonin in the brain. But it is much safer to eat foods containing DHA.

Your body cannot make sufficient amounts of DHA to supply your brain's needs. Therefore it is important that you get DHA in your diet on a daily basis. DHA is found in the following types of fish:

- Mackerel
- Salmon
- Sardines
- Tuna
- Herring
- Whitefish

Since DHA helps to create flexible brain structures, you can understand that people who have been diagnosed with Alzheimer's disease are twice as likely to have low levels of DHA in their blood. Conversely normal individuals who test with low blood levels of DHA have a two-thirds greater risk of developing Alzheimer's disease within ten years.

Fish oil or omega-3 fatty acids also prevent a buildup of substances called leukotrienes and cytokines, which produce inflammation. The inflammation caused by these agents can injure blood vessels and can also interfere with memory.

Fish really is "brain food"!

Polyunsaturated and monounsaturated fats

Polyunsaturated fats, which include safflower oil, sunflower oil, corn oil, and soybean oil, are damaging to the brain. Polyunsaturated fats are not the body-benefitting omega-3 fatty acids, but rather omega-6 fatty acids. These fats oxidize much faster than other forms of fat and create free radicals that can damage the brain. You should know that eating too much polyunsaturated fat can destroy DHA.

Monounsaturated fats are very good fats that help prevent bad cholesterol (LDL cholesterol, or low-density lipoprotein) from oxidizing. They can be found in the following foods:

- Extra-virgin olive oil
- Flaxseed oil
- Walnuts
- Avocados
- Almonds
- Macadamia nut oil

A simple way to improve your memory might be to stop using regular salad dressings and to switch to extra-virgin olive oil or flaxseed oil with vinegar.

Phospholipids

Just like omega-3 fatty acids, phospholipids are also important for optimal brain health. As the name implies, phospholipids are made of the combination of lipids (fats) and the mineral phosphorus. Phospholipids are found in high concentrations in the lining of practically every cell of the body, including brain cells. They help brain cells communicate and influence how well receptors function. Although present in many foods, phospholipids are found in higher concentrations in soy, eggs, and the brain tissue of animals. One of the most common phospholipids is phosphatidylserene (PS). PS is a brain-cell nutrient that rapidly crosses the blood brain barrier. PS boosts neurotransmitters in your brain that activate concentration, reasoning, and memory. This translates into your body having more ability to withstand the harmful effects of stress. Often these benefits will persist for weeks after PS is stopped.

BRAIN-HEALTHY EATING TIPS

- It's best to eat the protein portion of your meal first since this stimulates glucagon, which depresses insulin secretion and releases carbohydrates stored in your liver and muscles, helping to prevent low blood sugar.

- Eat slowly and chew well.

- Limit your starches to only one serving per meal. In other words, don't eat bread, pasta, potatoes, corn together at one meal. This elevates insulin levels. If you do go back for seconds, choose fruits, vegetables, and salads, but not starches.

- If you are craving a dessert, simply eliminate the starch or the bread, pasta, potatoes and corn and have a small dessert. However, be sure to have your protein and fat since this will balance out the sugar in the dessert. But don't make desserts a regular habit. Save them for special occasions such as birthdays, holidays, and anniversaries.

- Be sure that your diet has plenty of fiber. Fiber actually slows down the digestion and absorption of carbohydrates.

- Avoid alcoholic beverages, not only because alcohol is toxic to our bodies, but also because it triggers a tremendous insulin release and promotes storage of fat.

Common foods have insignificant amounts of PS, and the body produces limited amounts. Therefore, you need to obtain it in the form of a supplement. This brain nutrient helps maintain healthy cognitive function, thereby clearing up brain fog and mental confusion, helping restore lost trains of thought, and preventing the tendency toward misplacing items. In addition, phosphatidylserine supports cognitive function, emotional well-being, and behavioral performance by restoring cell membrane composition.[5]

Phosphatidylserine can be obtained in capsule form. Dosage is 300 milligrams daily, in divided doses. When taking PS, be patient. As with many natural supplements, it may take up to three months before you notice a measurable difference.

Keep memory sharp with ginkgo

Ginkgo trees are the oldest living trees on earth. The tree has long been associated with a long and healthy life. For centuries Chinese and Japanese traditions have used gingko leaves to support the brain, heart, and lungs. Today it can be obtained as a dietary supplement. The active components of gingko biloba, ginkgoheterosides and terpene lactones, enhance the flow of oxygen and blood to the brain and promote transmission of nerve impulses, thus supporting mental acuity. Gingko biloba offers nutritional support to the vascular system by sustaining the strength and elasticity of blood vessels and capillaries. In addition, it maintains healthy platelet function and acts as a free-radical scavenger.

> The following natural substances seem to help improve memory function:
> - Huperzine-A (club moss)
> - Periwinkle (vinpocetine)
> - Phosphatidylserine (PS)
> - Ginkgo
> - B vitamins
> - Vitamin E

Ginkgo cannot be obtained from foods, since the only source of it is the leaves of the ginkgo biloba tree, from which supplements are derived. Before taking Ginkgo supplements, be sure to heed the cautions (drug interactions, contraindications, dosages).

Sugar

Glucose, or sugar, is the brain's exclusive source of fuel. Therefore, getting enough is important. However, most Americans take in way too much sugar. The average individual consumes about 150 pounds of sugar per year.

Too much sugar will contribute toward lower mental functioning. Here's why.

Too much sugar in your blood will cause your pancreas to release insulin to lower the sugar level in your blood. Insulin is a hormone produced by your pancreas that regulates the amount of sugar in your blood. The body converts the food you eat into a form of sugar—glucose—and distributes it to the cells of the body through the bloodstream.

Each cell is a self-contained structure with a delicate environment. The cell membranes will not allow certain substances to enter without a "key" or "gatekeeper" to allow entrance into the cell. Insulin is the body's key that allows glucose to leave the bloodstream and enter a cell.

Under normal circumstances the pancreas efficiently manages the level of sugar in your blood day after day, year after year, without incident. Most people rarely think about their pancreas unless a problem develops.

High levels of sugar in your blood cause high levels of insulin to be released into your bloodstream. Maintaining these high levels for too long by regularly eating too much sugar and too many processed carbohydrates will cause your body to produce a regular oversupply of insulin. When this happens, your body can begin to become insulin resistant, which means that the insulin receptors on the body's cells—the gatekeepers or keys—stop functioning properly. This is usually an early stage of adult-onset diabetes. Too much sugar may cause your body's cells to begin refusing to allow sugar or glucose into the cells at all.

Remember that glucose is the brain's exclusive source of fuel. If you are becoming insulin resistant (in other words, if your insulin is not working effectively to allow the sugar into your cells), then your brain cells may not get enough glucose. It's like having a car without enough fuel to run. Since your brain uses sugar or glucose as fuel, your brain stops getting it if your cells stop receiving it. The result? Memory loss and clouded thinking.

Therefore, it's vitally important that you do not overload your body with sugary foods and carbohydrates that will elevate your insulin to unsafe levels.

Just as high blood sugar can impact mental functioning, low blood sugar can also have an effect. If brain cells do not have enough glucose, the mitochondria, which are the energy-producing portions of the brain cells, cannot produce enough energy. This can result in memory problems and mood swings. Such symptoms are commonly experienced by people with hypoglycemia who become irritable, foggy-headed, or agitated when they miss a meal.

Your brain needs to have an adequate and steady supply of glucose to function at peak performance. This is why your body works hard to maintain a fairly constant level of glucose in the blood in order to service the brain. But you can help your body keep your glucose levels fairly constant by eating every three to four hours.

PMS brain fog

Premenstrual syndrome affects a woman's brain and her ability to think clearly, to concentrate and learn, and to function effectively. For many women brain fog, or mental fog, is the worst part of PMS, outweighing anxiety, irritability, aches and pains, bloating, food cravings, and other annoying and debilitating symptoms that make their lives difficult each month.

"Brain fog" is a lighthearted way to talk about something that can cause a woman to make serious mistakes, reduce her resilience in the face of challenges, and prevent her from absorbing new information. Whether you are a student, a career woman, or a stay-at-home mom, the people around you may blame you for your lack of clarity and difficulty concentrating. They don't know that it's right before your period. This often becomes an unfortunate cycle; errors on the job, poor performance on school exams, and failing to keep up with the multiple requirements of home and family deal blow after blow to your self-confidence. And you may not realize at all that hormones are the cause of your difficulties. Your other PMS symptoms seem to take center stage.

Important tips for maintaining mental clarity

1. Maintain healthy sleep habits throughout the month: you know that when you have a bad night's sleep, you're more tired and irritable, and simply can't concentrate as well the next day. Many women experience some degree of insomnia in association with PMS or menopause, but maintaining healthy sleep habits that help keep you well rested throughout the month will help you cope with sleepless nights.

2. Exercise. A brisk walk is good for everything that ails you, including cloudy thinking.

3. Discover and avoid your food intolerances and sensitivities. This alone can clear the fog from your mind.

4. Stay regular. Just as food allergies can create brain-fogging chemicals in your bloodstream, so can constipation. One simple way to stay regular is to add one or two tablespoons of ground flaxseed to a serving of cereal or yogurt or vegetables. This will provide all-important fiber, along with lignans that may help prevent cancer and some important omega-3 fatty acids.

5. Junk the junk food. Like food allergens, junk food muddles your thinking by playing havoc with your brain chemistry.

6. Maintain stable blood sugar. Glucose (blood sugar) is your brain's fuel. When your levels go up and down, you feel woozy and energyless. Clear thinking goes out the window.

7. Adjust your schedule. If you experience monthly PMS or other hormonal shifts that make it hard for you to think, rearrange your obligations so that high-demand activities happen when you are feeling better. You don't have to be Wonder Woman (and even Wonder Woman must have to make hormonal and health adjustments from time to time).

Some degree of memory loss is inevitable, but it does not need to signal the end of a happy life. A woman who puts into place some brain-building measures will never regret it.

For God has not given us a spirit of fear, but of power and of love and of a sound mind. —2 Timothy 1:7, NKJV

Chapter 12
SLEEPLESSNESS AND INSOMNIA

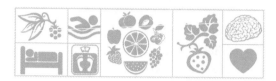

SWEET SLEEP—IT IS essential. Sleep experts tell us that while seven hours of sleep per night is the minimum amount needed, eight hours is still optimal. Certain regenerative processes within the body occur during sleep and do not take place during waking hours. It is only during rest that a person's bone marrow and lymph nodes produce substances to empower the immune system. Furthermore, it is during the beginning of your sleep cycle that much of the body's repair work is done.

Yes, sleep is vital. Yet because of busy lifestyles, women often find themselves burning the candle at both ends, staying up late and getting up early in the morning. According to the National Sleep Foundation:

> Women are more likely than men to have difficulty falling and staying asleep and to experience more daytime sleepiness at least a few nights/days a week. Research has shown that too little sleep results in daytime sleepiness, increased accidents, problems concentrating, poor performance on the job and in school, and possibly, increased sickness and weight gain.
>
> Getting the right amount of sleep is vital, but just as important is the quality of your sleep. Biological conditions unique to women, such as the menstrual cycle, pregnancy, and menopause, can affect how well a woman sleeps. This is because the changing levels of hormones that a woman experiences throughout the month and over her lifetime, like estrogen and progesterone, have an impact on sleep. Understanding the effects of these hormones, environmental factors, and lifestyle habits can help women enjoy a good night's sleep.[1]

Sad but true—sleepless nights
increase the speed of the aging process.

Lack of Sleep Impairs Performance

Let's say that a woman who needs eight hours of sleep per night gets only six. This two-hour sleep loss can have a major impact, including:

- Reduced alertness
- Shortened attention span
- Slower-than-normal reaction time
- Poorer judgment
- Reduced awareness of the environment and situation
- Reduced decision-making skills
- Poorer memory
- Reduced concentration
- Increased likelihood of mentally "stalling" or fixating on one thought
- Increased likelihood of moodiness and bad temper
- Reduced work efficiency
- Loss of motivation
- Errors of omission (making a mistake by forgetting to do something)
- Errors of commission (making a mistake by doing something but choosing the wrong option)
- Episodes of "microsleep" (brief periods of involuntary sleeping that range from a few seconds to a few minutes in duration)[2]

Sleep deprivation clouds the thoughts, changes the personality, and ages a woman faster than time itself. It costs nothing, but many women would pay just about anything for a night of sweet, sound sleep.

Elusive Sleep

Sleep can be elusive for a number of reasons. For women, the discomforts of PMS or hard-to-manage menstrual flow can shift in time to the hormonal changes at menopause, which bring hot flashes and night sweats. Other possible causes of sleeplessness include the use of decongestant medications, cold remedies, antibiotics, appetite suppressants, contraceptives, and thyroid medications. Deficiencies in potassium and the B vitamins, so common due to stress or chronic pain, may also be a factor in the poor sleep picture.

Especially for women, hormonal imbalances, sick children, daytime stress or anxieties, or pain can cause sleep deprivation to become a vicious cycle. After a woman suffers from several shortchanged nights for whatever reason, she may unintentionally aggravate her situation by eating poorly, avoiding exercise, and more. Her fatigue makes her accident prone. She makes poor decisions. Her relationships suffer. She catches the nearest virus and now she can't sleep because she's ill.

Many women in premenopause or menopause would love to be able to sleep as soundly as they did before they had children. Declining hormone levels may be responsible, as well as the fact that motherhood has conditioned them to become light sleepers. It doesn't seem to improve as children become teens, when both mothers and fathers may keep all-night vigils, waiting for their kids to return home safe and sound from their evening escapades.

CHECK YOUR REST QUOTIENT

- Sleep—I sleep soundly through the night, getting at least seven to eight hours of sleep nightly.
- Work—I minimize excessive work hours. I determine the time I will go home at the beginning of the day and stick to it.
- Rest—once a week, I take a day of rest in which I do not do my regular work and instead focus on rest, relationships, inspiration, and attitude.
- Vacation—at least once or twice a year, I take a vacation that allows me to slow down or get away from it all in order to relax and rejuvenate.

Symptoms of Sleep Deprivation

Drawn from the list above, the most common symptoms of sleep deprivation include the following. (Note that many of these symptoms can be related to disabling conditions, and the overlap of symptoms may make it difficult to determine if they are caused by sleep deprivation or the disability.)

- Tiredness
- Irritability, edginess
- Inability to tolerate stress
- Problems with concentration and memory
- Frequent infections
- Blurred vision
- Vague discomfort
- Alterations in appetite
- Behavioral, learning, or social problems
- Activity intolerance

Some suggestions to help you determine the cause of your sleep deprivation include talking to your health care provider and keeping a log that contains signs and symptoms, situations affecting your sleep, medications, diet, and so forth. Remember to take the log with you when you discuss your sleep problems with your health care provider.[3]

How do you think you're doing in terms of getting adequate sleep? You can take the following test to see if you are experiencing excessive daytime sleepiness as a result of less than adequate nighttime sleep.

Epworth Sleepiness Scale

In contrast to just feeling tired, how likely are you to doze off or fall asleep in the following situations? (Even if you have not done some of these things recently, try to work out how they would have affected you.) Use the following scale to choose the most appropriate number for each situation.

0 = Would never doze
1 = Slight chance of dozing
2 = Moderate chance of dozing
3 = High chance of dozing

Chance of Dozing	Situation
_____	Sitting and reading
_____	Watching TV
_____	Sitting inactive in a public place (i.e., theater)
_____	As a car passenger for an hour with no break
_____	Lying down to rest in the afternoon
_____	Sitting and talking to someone
_____	Sitting quietly after lunch without alcohol
_____	In a car while stopping for a few minutes in traffic
_____	Total score

A score greater than 10 is a definite cause for concern as it indicates significant excessive daytime sleepiness.[4]

Insomnia in Midlife Women

Decreasing estrogen levels have been linked to increasing irritability, depression, sleep deprivation, and loss of memory. No definitive studies have established estrogen loss as the cause, although women who have surgically lost their ovaries seem to experience these symptoms at a greater level than those who enter menopause gradually. Of course, hot flashes and night sweats can disrupt normal sleep patterns. Poor sleep in turn leads to irritability, depression, and poor concentration.

> Create an ideal sleeping environment: dark and peaceful, with comfortable bedding and *no television!*

Follow the advice in other chapters of this book for relief from hot flashes and other symptoms of menopause. You may need "something to help you sleep." Sleep aids can range from herbal (valerian root), to antihistamine (for example, Simply Sleep, Unisom, Tylenol PM), to prescription (brand names include Ambien, Lunesta, and Rozerem). (Note that prescription sleep aids can be troublesome in long-term use and require the supervision of a physician.)

If you are taking prescription sleep aids, you should know that sleeping pills impair calcium absorption, are habit-forming, and may paralyze the part of your brain that controls dreaming. Many times they can leave a person feeling less than rested and impair the clarity of daytime thoughts.

Adrenal Exhaustion

Even before menopause, many women complain of feeling stressed-out and "old." It can be hard to get up in the morning, because sleep seems inadequate. Everything seems like a chore, and it takes increased effort to accomplish everyday tasks. Salty foods appeal. Romance loses its appeal. It seems like viral infections hang on for months. Concentration is difficult, and memory is poor. Light-headedness makes even standing up difficult. However, often the after-dinner hours bring a "second wind," which can contribute to staying up too late at the expense of sleep. These are the classic symptoms of low adrenal function, or hypoadrenia, an often-misunderstood, unrecognized, and underdiagnosed condition that can smolder just below the surface.

Weighing less than a cherry and no larger than a prune in size, your two adrenal glands perch atop your kidneys. From this vantage point, they greatly affect the function of every single tissue, gland, and organ in your body. In addition, they also have a profound effect on the way you think and feel. Your energy, your endurance, and your very life depend heavily on proper adrenal function. A few decades of physical, emotional, and environmental stress take their toll, often resulting in a roll call of hypoadrenia symptoms: low blood pressure, fatigue, lethargy, low libido, electrolyte and fluid imbalance, and changes in body systems (fat metabolism and cardiovascular).

The body shape can begin to change to more of an "apple" due to excess fat distribution in the midsection.

People with low adrenal function live with a feeling of general unwellness. They often turn to coffee, teas, colas, chocolate, and other stimulants to keep their energy levels up long enough to make it through the day. Unfortunately these substances only tax the adrenal glands more, which creates an exhausting merry-go-round that is hard to stop. Low blood sugar is also a part of the hypoadrenic picture, as well as allergies, asthma, low immunity, and arthritic pain, not to mention mental health symptoms such as anxiety, depression, fearfulness, difficulty concentrating, confusion, and frustration. Over time hypoadrenia can lay the foundation for more serious health conditions, such as fibromyalgia, asthma, autoimmune disorders, diabetes, and respiratory infections.

After years of the stressful, life-changing events of adult life—raising a family, building a career, meeting health challenges and accidents, keeping up with financial needs, losing loved ones to death—no wonder our adrenal glands are affected negatively. They are affected by every kind of stress, including lack of forgiveness. And much like batteries that are drained each time a stressor affects our lives, if they are not recharged by resting enough, eating a proper diet, and getting enough exercise, they give up the fight. And if you continue to consume stimulants (caffeine, sodas, teas, and so forth), a meltdown is possible.

Stress can cause muscles to tense. Tense muscles can also occur in reaction to soreness in an affected area. Tension results in odd postures, and so does pain. Joint and muscle pain result. Pain causes mental stress as well, which increases the release of adrenaline. Ultimately this exhausts the body and mind. Depression occurs after the exhaustion phase, which again magnifies the discomfort. Serotonin levels drop as the action of the "feel good" brain chemicals is hindered. Sleep is disrupted by the pain, tension, and exhaustion, further inhibiting the body's ability to release natural mood elevators known as endorphins.

People who suffer from this condition will often say, "I feel like I am just existing" or "I don't know where I went." The condition itself makes it difficult to apply helpful solutions.

It is much harder to rebuild your system after a meltdown occurs than to prevent a crash in the first place.

Certain personality traits and lifestyle factors are common to persons with low adrenal function. (Note that having one or more of these traits or factors does not necessarily mean you have hypoadrenia.) They are:

- Perfectionism
- Lack of sleep
- Being driven
- Using stimulants
- Having a type-A personality

- Lack of leisure activities
- Keeping late hours
- Staying in no-win situations (which creates stress and frustration)

Premenopausal and menopausal women need to pay special heed. Around the age of fifty, a woman's adrenal glands are designated to do double duty, picking up the slack for the ovaries as they begin to shut down their production of sex hormones. If the adrenals are taxed and worn out, they cannot help smooth out the transition into menopause. This is why many type-A women experience an almost unbearable menopause, complete with severe anxiety, monster hot flashes, extreme fatigue, and more. These women are often prescribed Paxil, Xanax, and the like just to get them through these transitional years while at the same time sparing their families from dealing with "Mom and her emotional imbalances."

Besides unrelenting stress and a personality that seems ill-equipped to handle it, other factors that can worsen adrenal fatigue are long-term use of cortico-steroid drugs for asthma, arthritis, and allergies; too much sugar and caffeine in the diet; deficiency in vitamins B and C, and the simple onset of menopause.

A woman with hypoadrenia may or may not have these symptoms (and please note that these symptoms alone do not constitute a diagnostic tool):

- Severe reactions to odors or certain foods
- Recurring yeast infections
- Heart palpitations and panic attacks

- Dry skin and peeling nails
- Clammy hands and soles of feet
- Low energy and poor memory
- Chronic low back pain
- Cravings for salt and sugar

Besides forcing herself to *rest,* a woman can fortify her depleted adrenal glands by adding the following to her diet: brown rice, almonds, garlic, salmon, flounder, lentils, sunflower seeds, bran, brewer's yeast, avocados, wheat germ, and flaxseed.

The full spectrum of B vitamins are helpful. B complex comes in two standard doses: 50 and 100 milligrams. The 50 milligram dosage is the recommended daily dosage for people who are already taking a multivitamin that has B vitamins in it. One of the B vitamins, pantothenic acid, is known as an anti-stress vitamin, and it may also play a role in the production of adrenal hormones. It is very helpful in alleviating anxiety and depression because it fortifies the adrenal glands. In addition, you need pantothenic acid to produce your own natural pain relievers, such as cortisol. This is very important because pain often goes hand in hand with emotional depletion.

Vitamin C serves both a strengthening and protective function. Vitamin C is required for tissue growth and repair, healthy gums, and adrenal gland function, and it also protects against infections. Unless you are on an antidepressant or receiving cancer therapy, you can also try L-tyrosine, an amino acid that helps build the body's natural supply of adrenaline and thyroid hormones. It converts to L-dopa, which makes it a safe therapy for depression. L-tyrosine supports the production of catecholamine neurotransmitters, enhancing mood and cognitive function especially in situations involving stress or when dopamine, epinephrine, or norepinephrine levels require additional support.[5] L-tyrosine is most often used for stress reduction, anxiety, depression, and allergies, and it also aids adrenal function.

Overcoming Fatigue and Sleeplessness Naturally

In addition to the following suggestions, make sure you are getting your recommended daily amount of vitamin B complex and vitamin E.

Passionflower helps relax the mind and muscles. It is an anti-spasmodic, sedative, and non-drowsy sleep aid. Take 30 drops of tincture form or one 500 milligram capsule thirty minutes before bedtime. The herb valerian may be useful as a minor tranquilizer for anxiety-related sleep disorders.[6] Although it has a strong odor that many people object to, it can be taken as a tea (1 to 2 grams) thirty minutes before retiring, or taken in the form of the fluid extract (one-half to one teaspoon) or solid extract (250 to 500 milligrams). Some people may feel groggy or experience a "hangover effect" from valerian. (Warning: Do not combine valerian or passionflower with tranquilizers or antidepressant medications. If you are taking these medications, be sure to talk to your health care provider before you take any dose of valerian.)

In addition, many people recommend the following supplements as sleep aids:

- Hops—helps to induce sleep and is a safe and reliable sedative
- Melatonin—a natural hormone that promotes sound sleep
- DHEA—a natural hormone that improves the quality of sleep
- L-theanine—an amino acid that, if taken thirty minutes before bed, promotes deep muscle relaxation
- Calcium—has a calming effect and, when combined with magnesium, feeds the nerves
- Magnesium—relaxes muscles and, with calcium, feeds the nerves

- Inositol—enhances REM (rapid eye movement) sleep, the stage of deep sleep at which dreaming occurs

Take your calcium supplement at night to help
you sleep and to reduce leg cramps.

Aromatherapy is a safe, pleasant way to relieve stress, elevate your mood, and relax. The effects of aromatherapy are immediate and profound on the central nervous system. In addition, aromatherapy makes you feel good by releasing mood-inducing neurochemicals in the brain. Aromatherapy promotes relaxation, alertness, restful sleep, and physical relaxation, and it can increase energy. It works by stimulating a release of neurotransmitters once an essential oil is inhaled. Neurotransmitters are brain chemicals responsible for pain reduction and pleasant feelings. Sandalwood is an essential oil that is particularly good for sleep and relaxation.

Develop a regular sleep pattern. Reduce caffeine intake (especially late
in the day), reduce alcohol, and avoid eating large, fatty meals that
will keep you up at night. Try to aim for eight hours of sleep nightly.

When you are trying to reestablish a healthy sleep pattern, you must avoid caffeinated items such as coffee, tea, sodas, and chocolate. You should also avoid late-night eating. It has been said that sleep doesn't interfere with digestion, but digestion interferes with sleep. If you do eat late, choose a food that will promote relaxation such as plain yogurt (which is rich in sleep-inducing tryptophan), oatmeal (which tends to promote sleep), turkey, bananas, tuna, or whole-grain crackers. Try a cup of chamomile tea, which is considered to be a nerve restorative and helps quiet anxiety and stress. This is probably due to the fact that it is high in magnesium, calcium, potassium, and B vitamins. If you have trouble falling asleep, an evening routine can help you. But don't exercise late in the day. Try to maintain a regular bedtime, adjusting it no more than an hour on weekends.

Exercise and Sleep

A good goal for most women is to work out at least three times per week for thirty to sixty minutes. Any amount is better than none, though, and you need to start slowly. If you have not been exercising, you should consult your physician before beginning an exercise routine. Start with small changes such as taking the stairs, walking to work, or walking on your lunch break. Begin with ten minutes of moderate exercise, such as walking, each day, and then increase the amount of time and the intensity at which you exercise.

It is important to make exercise a habit so you are able to stick with it. Warm up with some light stretching for five to ten minutes to help prevent injuries. Stick to a regular time and keep a log of activities. Set goals, but don't get discouraged if you don't see changes immediately. Vary your routine so that you do not get bored. Find an activity you enjoy—you will be much more likely to stick with it if you are having fun.

GOOD SLEEP HABITS

The following tips about sleeping make sense for women of all ages:

- Go to bed and awake at the same time each day, even on weekends. (There is no way to make up for lost sleep.)

- Establish a daily cool-down time. One hour before bedtime, dim the lights and eliminate noise. Use this time for low-level stimulation activities such as listening to quiet music or reading nonstimulating material.

- Associate your bed with resting. Talk on the phone or surf the Internet elsewhere.

- Don't drink caffeinated drinks in the afternoon or evening. Caffeine's stimulating effects will peak two to four hours after consumption, but they can linger in the body for several hours.

- Don't eat dinner close to bedtime, and don't allow overeating. Sleep can be disrupted by digestive systems working extra hard after a heavy meal.

- Avoid exercise close to bedtime. Physical activity late in the day can affect your body's ability to relax into a peaceful slumber.[7]

There is a difference between being active and exercising. While it is true that you will burn more calories by leading an active life than a sedentary one, you have to get your heart rate up in order to get the most benefits from your exercise. Regular exercise can reduce your risk of heart disease, diabetes, osteoporosis, and obesity. Exercise keeps you flexible and makes it easier for you to move. The effects of aging are reduced, and your outlook is improved. Stress and anxiety are reduced, as is depression.

And even though you may feel tired after exercising, overall you will find that you have more energy and you will sleep better. Regular exercise will increase your metabolic rate so that even on the days you spend reading a book, you will burn more calories. Your body composition will change as you build muscle, which positively affects insulin and blood sugar control, lowering your risk for cardiovascular and other diseases. Exercise enables you to sleep better at night, and to have more energy when you want to be active.

Quality of Life

To recap: don't forget that lack of sleep robs your body of essential downtime necessary to rebuild vital organs and recharge your nervous system. People who return from a restful vacation will say they feel rejuvenated. Friends and coworkers will usually comment on how rested and relaxed they appear. Just think: if it is so evident on the outside, imagine what has taken place inside the body, mind, and spirit.

Your life expectancy can be extended substantially if you make sure that you are doing all you can to build and maintain your health. The foundation is simple: de-stress, get plenty of exercise, maintain healthy relationships, make healthy food choices—and sleep enough.

HE GIVES HIS BELOVED SLEEP

It is in vain for you to rise up early, to stay up late, and to eat the bread of hard toil, for He gives sleep to His beloved.

—PSALM 127:2

Chapter 13

FIGHT AGING BY RESTORING HORMONE BALANCE

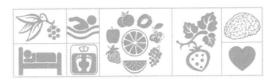

COMPLETING THE FIFTH decade of life can be an "aha" moment in which you celebrate and embrace with all that you have overcome and the milestones you have accomplished. Or depending upon how you have spent your younger years, reaching the big 5-0 can be an "oh, no" moment. In any case, this decade is a time of losses. We lose our hormones, our hair, and our car keys.

If you have stressed too much, lived on too little sleep, eaten poorly, failed to exercise, and burned the proverbial candle at both ends, you will be left with a shortened wick. In other words, your bank account of physical, emotional, and spiritual health can be seriously overdrawn at midlife, which can lead to a midlife meltdown. You may be aging faster than necessary in your body, mind, and spirit due to "sins of the past" coupled with the pressures of the present and the fear of the future.

Simply arriving at middle age often brings with it internal stress and such intense external pressure that life offers little or no joy. Physical symptoms such as overwhelming fatigue and lethargy are often a constant battle, enthusiasm for things once cherished is diminished, hope is dashed, and uncertainty is plentiful. A free fall occurs as our "safety net" of invincible youth gives way.

Assess Your Situation

In addition midlifers may grapple with aging parents and children leaving home for college (only to return overqualified and unemployed). Even the best of marriages go through a myriad of changes, and divorce is more common than not. For the first time in years, you and your husband will be forced to look closely at the strengths and weaknesses of your marriage. If you do not rediscover each other and develop new shared interests, you will not be able to replace with something meaningful the all-consuming work of child rearing and work.

If you are a single parent, having a supportive circle of friends becomes even more important, as well as having close family ties. You may decide to take advantage of new freedom from child-rearing responsibilities to make exciting new changes such as changing careers, taking classes, or dating. You may even remarry, deciding to risk the fact that both of you will by now have accumulated some life "baggage."

By midlife poor lifestyle and dietary habits in the past have set the stage for certain health conditions and degenerative diseases. The lack of a strong spiritual life becomes evident when you consider all the substance abuse or mood-elevating medications that are used in attempts to cope with all the difficult midlife issues. Recognizing that you are aging is unsettling—physically, relationally, emotionally, financially, hormonally, and more!

Many of the situations that occur at fifty are uncontrollable, and this is the time of life when you find out, maybe for the first time, that you are not in control. The good news is that midlife can be a turning point for those who will use it as such. It is time to take inventory of your life. It is the time to pay attention to the whispers that have been alerting you of the imbalances in your professional, personal, and family life, as well as your physical, emotional, and even financial health. It is a time to put your hands back on the wheel in terms of your life's course. It is a time to reflect on the past and what you have learned from it. It is the time to get rid of any baggage you are still toting on this earthly journey that may be weighing you down, such as debt, unforgiveness, anger, and personal relationships that take all your energy and rob you of being all you were meant to be.

Hormones are definitely not what they used to be. Both you and (if you are married) your husband are in a midlife transition. If both partners are going through the transitional years of menopause and andropause ("male menopause"), as is often the case, life together can be especially difficult, given the irritability and fatigue that hormonal decline can bring.

If you have children, midlife will bring empty-nest syndrome. Your children grow up, leave home for college, get jobs, get married, and start having their own children. An empty quietness fills the house, a reminder that a chapter in life has ended. The empty-nest syndrome affects women much more than men due to the fact that women are natural-born nesters. When the nest is empty, women must find something else to nurture. Many women need to take this opportunity to nurture themselves—before they begin the next chapter in their lives. It is a fact that both men and women are living longer these days. If you nurture yourself when you begin to notice the signs of aging, you can revitalize your mind, body, and spirit and redefine the aging process. If you are willing to do the work, this will help ensure that your upcoming "golden years" are truly that.

Finding Yourself on the Other Side

No doubt about it, midlife is a time of loss. We are losing our hormones. Our parents may be unwell or dying, and our children are leaving to begin their own lives. Strangely enough it is during this time of loss that many people find themselves again. Ask anyone who has experienced loss and is on the other side of the experience. Many times they will tell you that they were forced to return to the person they truly are. In other words, they no longer live their lives based upon others' expectations. They no longer live to please the world and other people, nor do they do things that they don't want to do. They have a stronger sense of self. They redefine themselves. Many have developed a strong prayer life during a season of loss. They emerge stronger, wiser, and more grounded than ever before.

The important thing is dying healthy—
not living the longest being sick.

By the time you have lived more than half of your life expectancy, you receive the gift of realizing that the real you represents more than your earthly frame. The aging process itself makes this inevitable, as physical changes accumulate and you see that you are not indestructible. This may be humbling, but that is a good thing if it encourages you, perhaps for the first time, to seek God and to develop and cement your personal relationship with Him. What a gift to discover that there is definitely a God who is more magnificent and loving than any person, place, or thing. This is a great blessing when being an active part of the sandwich generation takes a bite out of your life.

Changing Focus

Your priorities change, and the change is healthy. Instead of your focus being on career, child rearing, and other issues that consumed your younger years, longevity now holds the number-one position on your priority list. Instead of feeling competitive pressure to reach the top of the corporate ladder, you become more accepting and relaxed about your accomplishments, and you may begin to focus on retirement.

The marriages that survive midlife crises become stronger and more stable after weathering the financial, hormonal, and child-rearing storms common to all marriages.

The aging process and stress are constant companions that must be dealt with proactively on a daily basis.

If you are a young or middle-age woman, you can prevent many future problems by changing your habits now. If you are an older woman and are experiencing health issues, it is never too late to bring balance and harmony to your body. Aging is not a disease; it is a natural process. Most of the diseases that are normally associated with aging such as cancer, diabetes, digestive problems, depression, sexual dysfunction, and fatigue are not inevitable parts of growing older.

SELF-EXAM—SIGNS OF AGING

- Have you noticed brown spots on the back of your head or around your eyes and nose?
- Is it more difficult for you to lose weight?
- Do you have frequent indigestion, heartburn, or gas after eating a meal?
- Do you have insomnia?
- Do you have heart palpitations or chest pain?
- Do you have poor eyesight?
- Have you experienced hearing loss or ringing in the ears?
- Are you frequently constipated?
- Is your hair turning gray?
- Have you lost height?
- Is your skin becoming dryer or thinner? Are you noticing more moles, bruises, or cherry angiomas (red blood blisters)?
- Is your recovery time slow from a cold or flu?
- Do you have poor circulation?

The late comedian George Burns, who lived to be one hundred, summed it up beautifully: "If I knew I was going to live this long, I would have taken better care of myself."[1]

Living to old age should be a blessing and not a curse. All of these age-related disorders are mainly caused by lifestyle factors such as poor diet, lack of exercise, and exposure to toxins, along with genetic susceptibilities. Aging is accelerated by a lack of exercise. If you do not engage in regular exercise, you will increase your risk for almost every degenerative disease, including diabetes, osteoporosis, and heart disease. In addition, exercise helps to keep your blood sugar levels in the normal range.

The effects of stress play a role in the aging process as well. Women who endure long periods of intense stress are more likely to develop chronic disease. One of the biggest stressors for women is loneliness. One study found that lonely people have blood pressure readings that are as much as thirty points higher than people who are not lonely, and that more than half of people aged fifty to sixty-eight were experiencing some form of loneliness. You can do something about that! Instead of giving up or cutting back on social obligations, intellectual activities, sports, and other ways to connect with people, you can seek out new friends and activities that match your current capabilities.

How can you know whether the signs of aging you are experiencing are occurring more quickly than they need to occur? Take the previous quiz to help determine if you are aging faster than necessary.

Health Screenings for Every Woman Over Forty

When it comes to your health care, you may have the impression that age forty marks the beginning of midlife meltdown. The fact is, prevention and early detection of disease should be the cornerstone of your midlife wellness plan. Think of it as a screening evolution that began with the very first vaccine you received as a newborn. You should consider having the following health screenings. Think of this as your "Balanced Woman's Health Insurance Plan."

Dermatological (skin) exam. Like other illnesses that wait until you are older to rear their unattractive head, skin problems escalate at midlife. While it is important to keep an eye on any skin changes yourself, a good dermatologist is likely to see problems you might overlook. Your doctor will do a head-to-toe skin check, looking for irregular moles and other signs of skin cancer. Women ages forty and older should have this test once a year. Those with fair skin or who mistakenly assume a tan is as healthy as it looks may need to be on a more frequent schedule. Protect yourself; wear a hat and use sunscreen.

Colorectal cancer screenings. Starting at age fifty, all adults should have a fecal occult blood test annually and a sigmoidoscopy every three to ten years to check for polyps or cancerous lesions. Your physician may suggest a colonoscopy instead.

Total thyroxin test (T4). This blood test assesses thyroid function. Talk to your physician about getting the test around menopause.

Bone density test. You'll need a baseline test at menopause to detect osteoporosis or assess your risk for the disease. See chapter 9 for more information.

Clinical breast exam. Your physician should examine your breasts each year to look for lumps, swollen lymph nodes, and other irregularities. A baseline mammogram is recommended by age forty, followed by mammograms yearly.

Pap smear. You should have a pelvic exam yearly and a Pap smear (Pap test) at least once every two or three years (annually if you are at high risk for cervical cancer). You need a Pap smear even if you have had a hysterectomy or are postmenopausal. Pap tests were developed to detect cervical cancer, but they can also pick up infections, inflammation, and abnormal cells that may become cancer. Do not douche, use vaginal suppositories, foams, or medications at least two days before the test. Refrain from sexual intercourse for twenty-four hours. If you still have menstrual periods, schedule an appointment between the tenth and twentieth days of your cycle and never during a period. A stick, swab, or brush is used to dislodge a few cells from the cervical area, place them on a slide, and interpret them at a laboratory. Since the test is not 100 percent accurate, it is repeated if results are other than normal.

DOES YOUR THYROID GLAND NEED A BOOST?

Unrelenting fatigue, slow heart rate, cold hands and feet, moderate weight gain, swollen thyroid gland, hair loss, constipation, dry skin, poor memory, depression, and changes in personality—all are signs that your thyroid gland may need a boost. If any of these symptoms sound familiar, a simple blood test can determine if you need to take action and support your "metabolic pacemaker." Thyroid disease affects nearly fifteen million people, with most sufferers being women. Among women over the age of sixty-five, one in ten has early stage hypothyroidism. The reason doctors often miss so many cases of poor thyroid function is that the symptoms associated with thyroid disorder mimic the signs of aging. The range and severity of symptoms also vary greatly from one person to the next.

Glaucoma screening. Get this eye test beginning at age forty. Even if you have normal vision, you should get an eye exam every three to five years, and more frequently if you have any vision irregularities.

Electrocardiogram (ECG). You should get a baseline ECG by age forty. This painless test uses electrodes to record your heart's electrical impulses. The test evaluates heart function and can identify injury or abnormality.

Blood pressure screening. Blood pressure should be checked at least once every two years. If blood pressure is elevated, steps should be taken to control it; more frequent monitoring may be required.

Cholesterol test. If your LDL, HDL, triglyceride, and total cholesterol levels fall within the desirable range, this simple blood test, which helps assess your risk of cardiovascular disease, should be performed every five years.

Blood work. Especially as you reach your midlife years, your doctor should perform a formal assay (blood work) on you every year. Among other things, the results of your assay will help your health care provider determine a hormone-balancing plan tailored to your specific needs. An annual assay will serve as a guide to ensure that balance is achieved and maintained. This assay should determine your levels of the following:

- DHEA sulfate
- Progesterone
- E1, E2, E3 (estradiol, estrone, and estriol)
- T3
- T4 (thyroid panel)

- TSH (thyroid-stimulating hormone)
- FSH (follicular-stimulating hormone)
- LH (luteinizing hormone)
- Testosterone

Recognize the fact that enlisting a medical practitioner to order tests for you does not absolve you of responsibility. You must be aware of the tests your practitioner should be ordering. You need to have a general idea as to why and when they may be necessary—especially in light of your personal history. In this day of cost cutting, it is unlikely that your practitioner will add tests that are not necessary. But test results outside of a context are of minimal value. Do your homework and find out as much as possible about your family and your health history as a child. What serious illnesses have relatives suffered; what did they die from and at what age? Age is significant with breast cancer and heart attacks, because genetic risk will vary depending on when they occurred. Your own health history and lifestyle are relevant in analyzing and deciding what to do with test results.

It is never fun to discover you have a "risk" for a disease, nor is it easy to hear that some reparative action is in order. Baseline testing is likely to reveal that disease propensities exist. There is a difference between having a risk for a disease and having the disease itself, however. Differentiation between the two is important.

The actual danger you face and what you decide to do is equivalent to putting a rather challenging puzzle together. Test results, family history, personal health, philosophy about wellness, and available financial and medical resources must all fit together. Choosing to improve overall health by stopping smoking, losing weight, eating nutritiously, drinking plenty of water, exercising your mind and body daily, and working on a life in balance will not cause harm.

In contrast it could be harmful to take a prescribed drug or an herbal remedy simply because you have heard it might be protective. Before taking anything, be aware of the risk/benefit profile. Also think critically about the trade-off of drug therapy that is initiated to ameliorate risk rather than as treatment for an existing disease.

Finding Hormonal Balance

Aging itself causes a hormonal imbalance that may be a contributing cause of many diseases and ailments associated with aging, such as osteoporosis, loss of libido, depression, and coronary artery disease. Simply taking lots of vitamins will not make you feel better if you suffer from a hormonal imbalance, but you can endeavor to restore balance to your body as hormone levels decline by using bioidentical natural hormone supplementation.

Bioidenticals are hormone supplements that work with your body to enhance and reestablish your natural internal balance. Since they complement your natural hormones, your body accepts and uses them to reestablish your natural balance without the dangerous and uncomfortable side effects of synthetic hormones. Examples of bioidenticals would be natural estrogen or progesterone derived from plant sources such as soy or Mexican wild yam. Keep in mind the cautions regarding these foods mentioned previously. Or you may use herbs such as black cohosh and vitex.

BENEFITS OF MIDLIFE PROGESTERONE USE

Estrogen's Effects	Progesterone's Effects
Increases body fat	Helps use fat for energy
Increases salt and fluid retention	Acts as a natural diuretic
Increases risk of breast cancer	Helps prevent breast cancer
Decreases sex drive	Restores sex drive
Causes headaches and depression	Acts as a natural antidepressant
Impairs blood sugar control	Normalizes blood sugar levels
Increases risk of endometrial cancer	Prevents endometrial cancer
Reduces oxygen in all cells	Restores proper cell oxygen

Synthetic progestins, such as Provera, are not found in nature but follow the same hormonal pathways and bind to the same progesterone receptor sites. However, they do not act the same as natural progesterone, and they are not used as precursors for other hormones as is natural progesterone. Provera is the most popular progestin, which is a synthetic compound and is able to maintain the lining of the uterus.

Synthetic progestins can create many unpleasant side effects. When they unite with the same receptors as natural progesterone, they convey a different message to the cells. Side effects include fluid retention, breakthrough bleeding, blood clots, acne, hair loss, breast tenderness, jaundice, and depression. When synthetic estrogen and progesterones are combined, the adverse reactions may include a rise in blood pressure, PMS, changes in libido, changes in appetite, headaches, nervousness, fatigue, backaches, hirsutism (an increase in body hair), loss of scalp hair, rashes, hemorrhagic eruptions, itching, and dizziness.

Natural progesterone may help to protect you against breast cancer, osteoporosis, endometrial cancer, and fibrocystic breast disease. It acts as a natural antidepressant, and it may also improve your sex drive. Many middle-age women lack this valuable hormone, which may explain the midlife epidemic of anxiety, depression, and fatigue. Lack of progesterone may also be setting women up for potentially lethal diseases. Synthetic progesterones have similar protective effects as natural progesterone, however, as noted, they may produce many adverse reactions.

YAM IT UP

Yams and sweet potatoes are rich sources of DHEA. This important precursor hormone can become estrogen, testosterone, or progesterone as needed in the body. As we age, our body's level of DHEA drops, which hampers our antiaging defenses. But consuming sweet potatoes and yams on a regular basis guarantees high amounts of beta-carotene, vitamin C, protein, and fiber, as well as DHEA, which all work in symphony to provide energy and promote a vibrant life.

DHEA

DHEA (dehydroepiandrosterone) is a hormone that can be converted by the body to the hormones testosterone and estrogen. Levels of DHEA are naturally very high among teens and young adults but begin to decrease by the early thirties. The typical seventy-year-old has DHEA levels only about 20 percent as high as he or she had in the early twenties.

Scientists believe that the drop in levels of DHEA and the consequent drop of testosterone and estrogen may be related to many common age-related conditions, including diseases of the nervous, cardiovascular, and immune systems. Other conditions now believed to be related to diminished levels of DHEA and its end products include cancer, osteoporosis, and type 2 diabetes.

Restoring DHEA levels to those that naturally occur in younger adults may help slow the aging process and delay diseases of aging, such as heart disease, diabetes, and cancer. There is clinical evidence to back up this claim, including a study published in 2004 that showed reductions in abdominal fat and improvements in insulin sensitivity among older people who took DHEA for six months. A simple blood test can measure your DHEA levels. If they are low, the recommended dose for women is 15–20 milligrams per day.

PREMENOPAUSAL HORMONE BALANCE

In order to bring your estrogen and progesterone back into balance, try natural progesterone, which not only helps to restore balance, but also helps to regulate thyroid activity. Natural progesterone is essential for the production of cortisone in the adrenal cortex, and it helps prevent breast cysts. Natural progesterone helps combat premenopausal anxiety and mood swings. In addition it plays a very important part in the prevention and reversal of osteoporosis. Natural progesterone offers a woman all of these benefits without a high risk of the side effects of HRT. (The recommended dosage for women in premenopause is ¼ to ½ teaspoon, or 20 to 40 mg, applied to any clean area of the skin twice a day, morning and evening.

If you cannot find a doctor in your area who prescribes natural progesterone and natural estrogen, try a compounding pharmacy such as Women's International Pharmacy. You can contact them at their website, www.womensinternational.com, or at (800) 279-5708.

While DHEA has demonstrated antiaging benefits, new evidence supports DHEA's critical role in relieving depression, enhancing endothelial function, preventing atherosclerosis, increasing bone mass, slowing osteoporosis, improving insulin resistance, and even hastening wound healing.

Despite the life-extending and life-enhancing benefits of DHEA, it is not for everyone. People with hormone-dependent cancers such as breast, and uterine cancers should avoid its use. With that being said, there is an abundance of evidence that suggests that ensuring that you have optimal levels of this vital "prohormone" can help aging adults guard against many debilitating conditions once thought to be the inevitable consequences of aging. Again have your serum levels of DHEA tested by your health care provider. If you are in fact low, you may want to consider boosting your levels to the optimal range by taking a DHEA supplement.

MEASUREMENTS OF HORMONES			
Why?	How?	Who?	Results?
Measures estradiol, estrone, estriol, progesterone, and testosterone levels and their ratios of one to the other; follicular-stimulating hormone (FSH) and sex-hormone-binding globulin (SHBG) levels	Saliva or blood; urine not as accurate; five- or twenty-eight-day saliva avoids "snapshot" effect; time of menstrual cycle relevant	Pre- and perimenopausal women to rule out early menopause as a contributing factor to depression, weight gain, etc.; premenopause, to improve ovarian function if experiencing infertility, painful or erratic periods; premature menopause	Not much relevance in premenopause; possible baseline for comparison; FSH above 40 signals menopause; FSH = 20 signals symptoms. Premenopause results: preovulatory = 1.5–11.4 MIU/ml (milli international units per milliliter); ovulatory = 5.1–34.2 MIU/ml; postovulatory = 27.6–132.9 MIU/ml

Are You Menopausal?

Hormone tests can measure individual hormones of many types, including FSH, testosterone, estrogen, and progesterone. A good test includes FSH, estrogen, and progesterone, at the least. The test measures each one individually, which has certain clinical relevance. If FSH measures in a certain level, we can draw conclusions about menopause.

Too often women who consult a medical professional for issues of menopause expect and/or request that her "hormone" levels be tested. It proves difficult to convince her she might not benefit from the information derived. Because the nature of premenopause is one of great hormonal flux, capturing test results that mean something can be difficult.

Most women merely confirm what is an obvious certainty of menopause—that hormones are produced at lower levels and they are "estrogen dominant." This is because menstrual cycles at menopause often occur without ovulation. When an egg is not released, progesterone production is reduced. This is normal for menopausal women. The truth is there are no standardized baseline levels of reproductive hormones that are correct for all women. Nevertheless many women use such levels in combination with other factors to help confirm their menopausal state.

ESTROGEN METABOLISM ASSESSMENT			
Why?	**How?**	**Who?**	**Results?**
Measures the ratio and levels of 2-OH and 16-OH estrogen metabolites.	Either blood or urine; premenopause: days 19–25 of period; women on HRT or oral contraceptives: 8–10 hours after their last dose.	Anyone with estrogen-dependent health problems such as breast cancer, lupus, osteoporosis, and heart disease; women who want a baseline from which to monitor the effectiveness of dietary, lifestyle, and hormone therapies.	The imbalance of estrogen metabolites can lead to serious health problems, including cancer.

Comment: While this is an FDA-approved test, it is unlikely it will be on your local laboratory's panel. Yet this test is at least as valuable as measuring hormone levels, perhaps more so. Because metabolite production can be influenced by paying attention to diet and lifestyle, results provide a baseline that can give a woman motivation to begin or maintain positive intervention.

Aging and Intimacy

As a couple comes into their forties and fifties, they will notice certain changes happening to their bodies that will cause them to reevaluate their sex life. Many couples will wrongly conclude that they have reached an age when sexual activity is no longer possible or no longer desirable. With the average life expectancy now reaching deep into the eighties and nineties, to abandon sexual activity as one ages is to forfeit some of the best years of marital intimacy.

Certain myths about sex and aging persist. One myth is that sex isn't important as people get older. Other things in life such as companionship or recreational activity can keep the marriage together. Even grandchildren can be a source of common interest for an older couple. Sex is really something one does when he or she is younger or wanting a family. After decades it isn't such a big deal anymore.

The second myth is that sexual activity is supposed to fade away due to the process of aging. The human body naturally tends to stop being able to be sexually active, and the desire for sex is supposed to follow the ability to have it. Since God created our bodies, when our bodies no longer can do the things it used to do, that must be a signal that it is time to stop being sexually active. Otherwise God would have made us capable of staying at the same level sexually.

The third myth is that sex after a certain age is dangerous. Men, for example, may be afraid that they will have a heart attack while having sex. The fourth myth is more prevalent for women. Since they are getting older and may not be as attractive physically as they once were, they must not be sexually attractive to their husbands. If he still wants sex, it is just to satisfy his own needs and not because he still finds her attractive.

The final myth is that, with menopause and erectile dysfunction, it is just too much of a bother to stay sexually active. It is easier for everyone involved if the issue never comes up and married life moves on without it. The amount of work involved is not worth the rewards.

What can we say about these myths? One has only to look at the Bible to see that God did not intend for us to stop being sexually active as we age. Examples from the Old Testament show couples who were still intimate as they aged, Abraham and Sarah being the prime examples of enjoying sex in the "golden years."

Even at the age of sixty-five, Sarah was so beautiful that when she and Abraham went to Egypt, the powerful pharaoh selected her to come into his harem (Gen. 12:11–15). Even when Sarah was well into her eighties, Abraham made her lie about being his wife so he would not get killed because of her beauty (Gen. 20). Yet she was barren. By the time God enabled Sarah to conceive their son, Isaac, Sarah was well into her nineties and Abraham was a century old (Gen. 21:5).

There is no record in the Bible that God had to convince Abraham to have sexual relations with his wife—just that He would cause her to conceive. The fact that they could still have sex was a given!

Hormonal Realities

The myths may be untrue, but the reality is that sexual relations will not be what they used to be as you age. And hormones have more to do with the changes than any other factor, largely because hormones control or affect so many of the other factors.

Staying in good health is obviously a worthwhile goal even if you never have sex, but the reverse is equally true: if you want to stay sexually active, you have to stay in good health. Almost every disease will have an impact on our sex lives. Heart disease, diabetes, hypertension, obesity—all have a significant impact on a couple's sex life.

Besides erectile dysfunction in the man and reduced libido in both partners, the aging woman must contend with increasing vaginal dryness and resulting painful intercourse. This, however, does not need to put an end to intimacy. Local vaginal estrogen creams can restore natural lubrication to ensure that intercourse is not uncomfortable for the woman. Sometimes also, vaginal surgeries are necessary to maintain a properly functioning vagina.

Women, take note: it is a biological fact that men reach orgasm much faster than women. This wide disparity has often left women without their fair share of orgasmic experiences. And because most women do not expect to achieve orgasm each time, the disparity is often left unmentioned. But now with age comes the great equalizer. It is as if God has remembered the woman and given to her the gift of time. Because it will now take the man longer to achieve and maintain an erection, the process cannot be rushed, as it once might have been when her husband was younger or when she was tired from the kids and just wanted to "get it over with." Now sexual intercourse is an experience that must be lingered over. It is all about the journey and not just the destination. This is when sex becomes intimate and not simply a race to the finish. And because the house is not filled with little children or demands of work, there is more time available to really explore each other and discover what brings each one pleasure.

The man must now learn to be creative and give his wife pleasure regardless of the ability he still possesses to have vaginal intercourse. Foreplay is now the most important thing, and this gives his wife the much-needed time she needs to be fully aroused and orgasmic.

Well Worth It

Getting older is challenging to be sure, but rewarding as well. The words of the late Scottish theologian and broadcaster Carl Bard can apply not only to sexual intimacy in later life but to all of the challenges of the aging process: "Though no one can go back and make a brand-new start, anyone can start from now and make a brand-new ending."[2]

Chapter 14

FOODS ESSENTIAL TO WOMEN'S HORMONE HEALTH

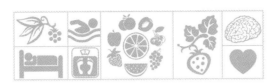

IT WOULD BE impossible to minimize the role that good nutrition plays in your overall health and body balance. The nutrients you consume each day in every bite of food you take are what give you energy to do your work and to empower your body with vibrant health.

Your body uses nutrition to build, maintain, and repair your tissues. Nutrients empower your cells to relay messages back and forth to conduct essential chemical reactions that enable you to think, see, hear, smell, taste, move, breathe, and eliminate waste. Is good nutrition crucial to body balance and vibrant health? You bet it is! But getting reliable information about nutrition can be a challenge.

This chapter focuses on the important role nutrition plays in supporting a woman's health. Good nutrition is the foundation of healthy cell function; it helps balance hormones, provides antiaging benefits, aids the production of energy, and protects from disease.

Many women neglect to nourish their bodies with life-giving nutrients because they are so involved with caring for others that they fail to devote their attention to healthy dietary practices for themselves. This chapter will educate you on what foods are best for your personal health and well-being. Once you apply these recommendations, you will be able to make informed dietary choices that will in turn help you to look and feel younger and, of course, be healthier. All women may share the same basic physical makeup, but each individual is as unique as her thumbprint when it comes to her specific nutritional needs.

Many factors combine to determine your individual nutritional needs, including:

- The amount of stress you experience and how you manage it
- How your hectic lifestyle depletes your nutritional storehouse
- What your dietary habits are

Nutrition is not boring! God doesn't intend for you to live your life eating bland, undesirable food. He has created the earth with a banquet of tempting and delicious choices not only to satisfy your taste buds, but also to support your health in every way as well. The Garden of Eden was a place where Adam and Eve feasted on a banquet of natural delights prepared by their loving Creator. They were truly and wonderfully blessed. Everything they ate in that exotic place was not only genuinely delicious, but it was also completely nourishing to their bodies.

Think about Adam and Eve and the Garden of Eden as you consider reestablishing your eating habits to help your body to regain the natural balance that was created by God for you to enjoy. To keep from becoming sluggish and estrogen-dominant, eat the following whole, fresh natural foods:

- Fruits
- Vegetables
- Whole grains
- Legumes (beans)
- Nuts and seeds

Stay close to the Garden of Eden when you make your selections. In other words, the more processed and man-made an item is, the more likely it is to throw your body out of kilter hormonally. In practical terms that means you should limit the following:

- Sugar
- Refined, processed carbohydrates such as white bread
- Instant potatoes and white rice
- Hydrogenated, saturated fats
- Too much polyunsaturated fat

This doesn't mean that you have to deprive yourself of an occasional sweet treat. Just try to be sure that most of your diet choices are close to the garden, which means they are whole, fresh, unprocessed, and completely natural. By carefully limiting the above foods, you should be able to balance your estrogen level as well as your cortisol level, thus relieving many PMS and menopausal symptoms.

Seek Out Phytoestrogens

Although you want to shun foods that are packed with synthetic estrogens (xenoestrogens), there are natural estrogenic foods that will actually greatly help you. These are called phytoestrogens. Phytoestrogens are found in some plants, and eating them can really help to get you hormonally balanced. Foods highest in plant estrogens include:

- Soy (natural, organic, non-GMO is best)
- Flaxseed
- Flaxseed oil

- Whole grains
- Parsley
- Fennel seeds
- Celery

Plant-derived estrogens help to balance out the estrogen in your body. If you have high amounts of estrogen, the plant estrogens will lower the estrogens. But if you have low estrogens, the plant estrogens will, by binding to the estrogens, actually raise and balance the estrogen levels. So phytoestrogens work both ways to give you hormonal balance.

Plant estrogens bind to estrogen receptors, but these plant estrogens are only about one-hundredth as strong as estrogen. Although you might think that eating plant estrogens might increase the amount of estrogen in your body, the effect is usually the opposite. Since many women with premenopause and PMS also have estrogen dominance, here's what happens. Your body receives the milder phytoestrogen, which binds to the estrogen receptor and tends to reduce your high estrogen level. That's why Oriental women who eat diets with a lot of phytoestrogens experience very little PMS. On the other hand, if your estrogen level is too low, the phytoestrogens will also bind to the estrogen receptors, causing an increase in estrogenic effect. These marvelous foods work hard to help your body balance your hormones.

The role of phytoestrogens as adaptogens—estrogen agonist and antagonist—means they involve themselves in different signaling and gene processes. Research confirms that increased isoflavone consumption leads to favorable metabolite ratios and decreased estrogen production. The following are favorable effects some of these nutrients provide:

Resveratrol. Resveratrol is found in many plants but is especially plentiful in grapes. It has its own special estrogen-modulating effects that lower breast cell proliferation and influence circulating estrogen.[1] New studies suggest grape juice has plenty of healthful properties should you not care to imbibe your medicine as red wine.[2] Lignans (found in flaxseeds, the bran layer of grains, beans, and seeds) and isoflavones (like soy and red clover) are converted in the colon to a biologically active form that in turn affects the production of hormones. Prompting a shift to 2-OH metabolites (good estrogen) is one of the most important things soy does. The presence of appropriate bacteria in a favorable balance is an essential part of the metabolic work. A person who has eaten soy for a lifetime is apt to have the proper ratio of bacteria and might gain significantly more than someone who has added soy to their diet only recently. In other words, it is not only what you eat, but also the mechanism to convert the food into a usable, effective form that is important.

Biologically active folate. Genetic variations can make you more susceptible to producing 4-OH or 16-OH metabolites ("bad" estrogen). Low levels of B vitamins (B$_6$, B$_{12}$, and folate) interrupt proper estrogen detoxification, resulting in increased estrogen. A significant percentage of the population have problems utilizing B-vitamin folate (folic acid), placing them at risk for higher levels of homocysteine and consequent peril for stroke and cardiovascular disease, depression, Alzheimer's, and colon and breast cancer. The problem is solved with biologically active forms of folate (5-formyltetrahydrofolate and 5-methyltetrahydrofolate).

Soy Food Products

The isoflavones in soy are the primary phytoestrogens that your body needs. One cup of soy is equivalent to a regular dose of Premarin. Whole, natural soybean products actually contain higher amounts of isoflavones than other soy protein products. Therefore choose soy flour or whole soy products rather than soy proteins in order to get your phytoestrogens. Or you may take a supplement containing approximately 50 milligrams of isoflavones per day. The isoflavone genistein is the primary phytoestrogen in soy. (See "Dark Side of Soy" for cautions and recommendations for consuming soy for greatest health benefit.)

Don't know tofu from tempeh? Here are some of the most common soy foods, along with a few suggestions for using them:

Soy flour—Made from roasted, ground soybeans, soy flour can be used to replace some of the wheat flour used for baking. Nutritionists advise buying defatted soy flour, which contains less fat and more protein than the full-fat variety.

Tempeh—These chunky, tender cakes are made from fermented soybeans that have been laced with mold, giving them their distinctive smoky, nutty flavor. You can grill tempeh or add it to spaghetti sauce, chili, or casseroles.

Tofu—A creamy white, soft, cheeselike food made from curdled soy milk, tofu can be used in virtually anything from soups to desserts. You will find soft and firm varieties of tofu at most supermarkets in the produce section.

Other soy foods are available at specialty and health food stores.

You may have heard that Japanese women have few difficulties and symptoms of menopause. Their incidence of hot flashes and night sweats is significantly lower than among Western women. In a cross-cultural sample with over eight thousand Massachusetts women and thirteen hundred Canadian women, twelve hundred Japanese women ages forty-five to fifty-five were compared. Medical anthropologist Margaret Lock reported that these Japanese women have sociological and biological factors such as diet that lower the symptoms of menopause. Other researchers have also suggested that the Asian diet with higher quantities of phytoestrogens lessens the symptoms of menopause.[3]

If you want to add more soy to your own diet, just be careful that you're not allergic to soy products—some women must avoid them.

> ### ARE YOU DRINKING ENOUGH WATER?
>
> Do a simple urine test: if your urine color is dark yellow, start drinking more water. You will know that you are adequately hydrated when your urine becomes a pale straw color.

What Should You Eat?

It never hurts to be reminded about which foods are genuinely good for you. Does your daily and weekly diet include some foods of all of these types?

Fresh fruits and vegetables

Fruits are nature's way of smiling. They have been referred to as "nature's candy." They are wonderful system cleansers. They are high in vitamins and nutrition, and have a naturally high water and sugar content that speeds up your metabolism to release wastes quickly.

Natural fruit sugars are easily transformed into quick, nonfattening energy that speeds up your metabolism. This is true for fresh fruits only. Fresh fruits should be eaten before noon for best energy conversion and cleansing benefits. Fruits offer you a wonderful source of potassium, calcium, magnesium, and vitamin A. Vitamin A is an important player in the prevention of many types of cancer and safeguards against cardiovascular events such as stroke and heart attack. It is also very important for clear vision and strong immunity. Potassium helps to regulate your body's fluid balance. Women with low potassium levels often have low stamina and fatigue easily.

Citrus fruits such as oranges, lemons, and grapefruit are high in vitamin C. Vitamin C has antioxidant activity and works synergistically to help recycle vitamin E. Vitamin C is also found in berries and green vegetables such as asparagus, broccoli, spinach, turnip greens, and dandelion greens. You should try to have three to five servings of fruit per day.

The most amazing fruit of all is the pomegranate. The pomegranate represents longevity and immortality in many ancient cultures. They have long been used in folk medicine around the world to treat cuts, sore throats, diarrhea, gum disease, and infections. Hippocrates used them for treating fevers. But today's research shows that it can really help prevent the most common health problems associated with aging, particularly heart disease. This truly amazing fruit addresses several aspects of heart disease, including atherosclerosis, blood flow, LDL oxidation, and high blood pressure. Laboratory research suggests that it may also be effective in cancer prevention, diabetes, neurological health, infection, and osteoarthritis.

Today the pomegranate is widely recognized for its antioxidant properties. Studies show that the pomegranate has more antioxidant power than any of the foods typically recommended as antioxidants, including blueberries, cranberries, red wine, and green tea. It is also more powerful acting than the common antioxidants vitamins A, C, and E. Pomegranates' antioxidant properties are attributed to its high content of soluble polyphenols, including a tannin called punicalagin.[4]

Most of the studies on the pomegranate have focused on its effect on heart disease. Clinical studies in humans have focused on the pomegranate's ability to prevent and treat atherosclerosis, diabetes, osteoarthritis, and cancer. A few studies have also documented the pomegranate's antibacterial and antiviral effects.

Some studies on the health benefits of pomegranates have explored their ability to stop and even reverse the buildup of plaque in arteries. These studies show that pomegranates offer significant health benefits for people at risk for heart disease. It has been suggested that pomegranates combat atherosclerosis by stimulating paraoxonase (PON) enzyme activity and HDL-associated protein. Animal studies show that polyphenols inhibit LDL oxidation and reduce atherosclerosis, thus reducing the risk for cardiovascular problems such as heart attack and stroke.

In addition to its cardiovascular protection, pomegranates offer help for osteoarthritis by inhibiting cartilage breakdown.[5] Researchers have identified two anti-dementia components in pomegranates: ellagic acid and punicalagin. Both of these components seem to inhibit a serine protease associated with dementia.[6]

When you add in all of the other benefits, which include improved immune functioning, neurological health, and protection against cancer and osteoarthritis, you can see how truly amazing the pomegranate really is! One fruit has it all; this brilliant red fruit can help prevent and reverse heart disease, help prevent dementia, and inhibit the cartilage breakdown associated with osteoarthritis.

You may have heard that it's the deepest-colored fruits and vegetables that carry the most nutritional benefit. By and large it is true. For example, red foods are lycopene-rich "superfoods." Lycopene is found in tomatoes, carrots, pink grapefruit, watermelon, apricots, and strawberries. High consumption of lycopene foods will reduce the risk of heart attacks.

Carotenoids are usually orange foods, but may also include dark green vegetables. They include carrots, watermelon, tomatoes, cantaloupe, pink grapefruit, sweet potatoes, squash, and spinach. Carotenoids may lower the risk of developing cancer and are very important in immune function.

And yes, you need to eat your broccoli. You need other cruciferous vegetables too such as cauliflower, cabbage, brussels sprouts, and kale. They have potent phytonutrients that are important in helping to prevent breast cancer. It is known that dietary intake of indole-3-carbinol (broccoli, cabbage, and other cruciferous vegetables) is protective because of its ability to influence positive liver function to excrete estrogen and to promote good estrogen metabolites. If you prefer your vegetables in pill form, two different extracts from cruciferous vegetables known as indole-3-carbinol and diindolylmethane (DIM) are roughly equivalent to eating two pounds of broccoli.

In addition, you will be healthier if you eat grass—really! Green foods that are high in chlorophyll include spirulina, chlorella, blue-green algae, barley grass, wheat grass, and alfalfa. These unusual vegetables contain almost every mineral and trace mineral necessary for human survival. They also cleanse our bodies of toxins and poisons and protect them from the damaging effects of these toxins.

Whole grains

A healthy diet contains three or more servings of whole grains each day. Whole grains such as oats, rye, millet, amaranth, quinoa, barley, whole-grain breads and pasta, and buckwheat provide fiber, protein, carbohydrates, fats, a wealth of minerals, B-complex vitamins, and other vitamins and lignans, which help with many reproductive problems.

Whole grains can help lower your total cholesterol by binding to it and helping to eliminate it from your body. Millet, in particular, is helpful for alkalizing the stomach and is acceptable for women who have wheat allergies and candida yeast overgrowth. Quinoa is gluten free. Oats are excellent fiber grains that help to lower cholesterol and promote regularity. Buckwheat is a non-wheat grain. Barley is a low-gluten flour with a sweet malty taste. Amaranth is an ancient Aztec grain-like seed that contains high-quality protein. Whole grains also serve women well because the fiber they contain binds to the estrogen that their bodies are trying to discard and makes sure that it is eliminated. In addition, the complex carbohydrates found in whole grains stabilize levels of serotonin, which provides a calming and relaxing function.

Legumes

If you are trying to reduce your consumption of animal protein, turn to legumes such as lima beans, pinto beans, garbanzo beans, navy beans, lentils, peas, and soybeans. All are great sources of fiber and complex carbohydrates. When you consume them along with whole grains, you create the same balance of amino acids that is equivalent to protein. Legumes are rich sources of B vitamins. If you combine them with whole grains and leafy vegetables, you are ensuring that your body is receiving inflammation-fighting essential fatty acids.

Nuts and seeds

Nuts and seeds are little storehouses of nutrition complete with omega-3 and omega-6 fatty acids, B-complex vitamins, and a plethora of minerals. The really great thing about them is that they help keep your skin supple and moist. This includes vaginal and bladder mucosa during your perimenopausal/menopausal transition and beyond!

Almonds, pecans, walnuts, sunflower seeds, pumpkin seeds, sesame seeds, and flax-seeds all offer you a bounty of benefits. You can sprinkle them on salads and whole-grain cereals. They make a great garnish for fruit salads too! Try to have a quarter cup of seeds or nuts several times a week.

Vitamins, minerals, spices. In the laboratory vitamin E has been shown to inhibit growth of breast cancer cells. Antioxidants such as green tea and D-limonene (from citrus fruits) prevent the formation of very reactive breakdown products of estrogen, important because they directly and negatively affect DNA. And research confirms that naturally occurring spices such as curcumin from the curry spice and turmeric, a member of the ginger family, can be effective in protecting against environmentally toxic estrogens that stimulate growth on receptor positive and negative breast cancer cells. They also enhance detoxification.

GIMME THE CHOCOLATE!

Most women crave chocolate during their "time of the month." They tend to feel better after eating something "chocolatey." The reason they crave chocolate is because their bodies are deficient in magnesium, and chocolate is a source of magnesium.

Magnesium is important for breakdown and excretion of estrogen, which is especially important for women in midlife. When you are chronically stressed, you can become deficient in magnesium even if you consume magnesium-rich foods on a daily basis. When you are exposed to continuous stress—perhaps from taking care of an elderly parent or dealing with hormonal issues, teenagers, financial problems, marital problems, or anything else that this phase of life brings your way—you become irritable and easily fatigued, and you lose your ability to concentrate. Your blood pressure may begin to creep up because adrenaline levels increase in your blood.

It is under these conditions that magnesium is released from your blood cells and goes into your blood plasma. From there it is excreted in the urine. A study in France found that this stress-induced depletion of magnesium was more dramatic in those with type-A personalities who were competitive and known to be more prone to heart disease. Some researchers suggest that this depletion of magnesium among type-A individuals may be the primary reason they carry an increased risk of heart attacks. It is also interesting to note that when an individual suffers a heart attack, magnesium is administered immediately.

Magnesium helps to regulate heart rhythms and thins the blood. Another benefit is the ability of magnesium to relax arteries, thereby lowering blood pressure.

Most Americans consume diets that fail to meet even the government's minimum recommended dietary allowance for magnesium. Most troubling is the inadequate intake among individuals who develop heart disease. In addition to adding the following foods to your diet, you can supplement with up to 400 milligrams of magnesium at bedtime. Magnesium-rich foods include:

- Almonds
- Bananas
- Blackberries
- Black-eyed peas
- Broccoli
- Dates
- Green beans
- Kasha
- Millet
- Navy beans
- Shrimp
- Soybeans (natural, organic, non-GMO is best)
- Tuna
- Watermelon
- Fiber

Making sure that your diet has enough fiber is also very important for controlling PMS and premenopause symptoms. Fiber helps to eliminate excess estrogen through the colon. It will unite with estrogen in the GI tract and prevent it from being reabsorbed back into the blood stream. High-fiber foods also help to lower the glycemic index and thus help to break you out of that awful cycle of eating sugar and craving starches. Foods high in fiber include:

- Beans
- Legumes
- Peas
- Lentils
- Fruits
- Whole grains (sprouted or gluten-free)

(Have you noticed a definite overlap in the types of foods that should be part of your diet? Many of them carry multiple benefits.)

Water

Water is an essential part of good health, making up 70 percent of your body weight. Diets that promise quick weight losses are really eliminating water or muscle, since only one or two pounds of fat cells can be lost per week. When you are in short supply of water, your body releases a hormone that causes you to retain water and sodium. You should consume half your body weight in ounces of water every day to ensure you are properly hydrated.

ADD LIFE TO YOUR YEARS
WITH GOOD NUTRITION

- Avoid fried foods, red meat, too much caffeine, and highly spiced and processed foods.
- Eat fresh seafood at least twice weekly for thyroid health and balance.
- Nuts, seed, beans, fiber, and essential fatty acids are living nutrients.
- Fresh fruits and vegetables are enzyme-rich and full of vitamins, minerals, and fiber.

Limited Access

By limiting your consumption of certain foods, you won't undo all the good of the healthful and nutritious foods you eat.

Sugar

Women who eat more sugar tend to experience more PMS and menopausal symptoms. If you eat high-sugar foods and processed carbohydrates, your blood sugar will rise along with a corresponding rise in insulin. But when insulin rises, it causes your blood sugar to plummet even lower than it was when you first started eating. Now a release of adrenaline and cortisol is triggered that will tend to cause an imbalance of progesterone, thus leading to unwelcome symptoms.

You can see what a vicious cycle this is. The insulin your body releases to bring down sugar will actually make you think you are craving more sugar. When you eat more sugar or highly processed carbohydrates, the cycle starts all over again. One of the many losers in this trap is your hormonal balance, because each time your sugar rises and drops, your hormones are also directly affected.

That's why it is critically important that you drastically limit all sugars and highly processed carbohydrates such as white bread, rice cakes, and cereals.

High sugar intake is also known to play a negative part in a host of our most common diseases, including hypoglycemia, heart disease, high cholesterol, obesity, eczema, psoriasis, dermatitis, gout, yeast infections, and tooth decay. Sugar is addictive, affecting the brain first by offering you a false energy lift that lets you down lower than when you started.

PERILS OF SUGAR

Mental and emotional signs of too much sugar:

- Chronic or frequent bouts of depression with manic depressive tendencies
- Difficulty concentrating, forgetfulness, or absentmindedness
- Lack of motivation, loss of enthusiasm for plans and projects
- Increasing independence, inconsistent thoughts and actions
- Moody personality changes with emotional outbursts
- Irritability, mood swings

Brain and body symptoms associated with excess sugar consumption:

- Anxiety and panic attacks
- Bulimia
- Candidiasis, chronic fatigue syndrome
- Diabetes or hypoglycemia
- Food addiction with loss of B vitamins and minerals
- Obesity
- Menopausal mood swings and unusual low energy[7]

In times of stress, depression, and anxiety, women often reach for sugar. This is especially detrimental to your brain and body function. In addition, excessive sugar consumption has been shown to suppress your body's immune response. If you are consuming too much sugar on a daily basis, you may be setting yourself up for low blood sugar. Many women who suffer from anxiety and depression also have to deal with hypoglycemia.

> ## TOO SWEET FOR HER OWN GOOD
> Too many sweets or carbohydrates can contribute to recurrent yeast infections. Diabetes also raises the sugar content of the vagina and promotes the growth of yeast. If your diet is high in sugar, cut out refined sugars altogether, and you will see a dramatic improvement.

Hold the salt

Lowering your salt intake is vital to your health. And since many PMS and premenopause symptoms are related to water retention, watching your salt intake can really make a difference.

Eating too much salt increases water retention, abdominal bloating, and edema. These common symptoms of premenopause and PMS are often caused by elevated cortisol and aldosterone levels. By decreasing your salt intake, most of these symptoms can be completely relieved.

Lower your salt by limiting high-sodium foods, which are mainly processed foods, and by eating more fresh fruits and vegetables. And be sure to keep the salt shaker off the table!

Then there's junk food

We are a junk food generation. What would have happened if Adam and Eve had been given junk food? Would they have eaten it? Would they have liked it? Probably not. As a matter of fact, when you get accustomed to giving your body plenty of whole, natural foods, you may begin to look at junk foods as not being real food at all!

Therefore, the Garden of Eden principle really applies to junk food. To live above the miserable symptoms of PMS and menopause, drastically cut down on the amount of junk food you eat.

Junk foods are high in sugar and refined, processed carbohydrates, which stimulate insulin release. This leads to the release of adrenaline and cortisol, which causes an imbalance in progesterone. As cortisol levels rise, they will eventually cause a decrease in progesterone levels.

Other dietary health robbers

The following foods have little or no place in a body-balancing program because they offer little if any nutritional benefit and may even leach many valuable nutrients from your body.

Caffeine. Caffeine stimulates the release of stress hormones, which will increase any feelings of nervousness or anxiety you may have as well as steal valuable nutrients from the rest of your body that are needed to feed your stressed nervous system. In addition, caffeine triggers panic and anxiety symptoms, reduces absorption of iron and calcium, worsens breast pain, increases the frequency of hot flashes, and acts as a diuretic, speeding the elimination of valuable minerals and vitamins you need. It increases acid production in the stomach and raises blood levels of cholesterol and triglycerides. Slowly wean yourself off caffeine by reducing your daily intake until you are caffeine-free. There are wonderful decaffeinated teas and beverages to choose from.

You can help balance your hormones by avoiding the following:

- Junk foods
- Sugar
- Processed foods
- Caffeine
- Alcohol
- Fried foods
- Margarine

Instead, select foods that are nutritionally healthy for you. Choose:

- Fresh fruits
- Fresh vegetables
- Lean meats
- Whole grains (sprouted or gluten-free)
- "Good" fats (seeds, nuts, olive oil, avocados)

Dairy. Many women who complain of fatigue, bloating, depression, intestinal gas, nasal congestion, postnasal drip, and wheezing may suffer from a food sensitivity, and most often the culprit is dairy. Dairy products are one of the primary sources of food allergies in the standard American diet. Delayed reactions such as mood swings, dizziness, headaches, and joint pain can occur. Another important consideration is lactose, which is the predominant sugar in milk and cannot be digested by many women. The good news is that there are wonderful dairy substitutes that are full of calcium and are easy to assimilate. Try rice milk or almond milk; try sorbet or other frozen desserts made from rice milk. Make smoothies with rice milk or almond milk. Try almond or rice milk cheese. Your body will quickly let you know that you have made a healthier choice. Watch all of your allergic symptoms disappear in about seven to fourteen days.

Fats and Hormones

The two main hormones made by the ovaries—estrogen and progesterone—are two of the steroid hormones in the body. Steroid hormones actually come from cholesterol, and most of the steroid hormones are very similar in shape. However, they have extremely different effects. The steroid hormones include progesterone, estrogen, pregnenolone, DHEA, androstenedione, testosterone, cortisol, aldosterone, and others.

Since all of these steroid hormones are made from cholesterol (animal fat—i.e. meats, whole milk, egg yolks), it is critically important never to go on a strict no-cholesterol or a no-fat diet. If you eliminate all cholesterol foods and fats from your diet, you may develop a hormone imbalance since all of the steroid hormones come from cholesterol.

Oils (fats) to avoid

Hydrogenated oils and partially hydrogenated oils are probably the most dangerous oils that you can consume. Avoid or decrease hydrogenated oils and most heat-processed vegetable oils in your diet. Hydrogenated oils and partially hydrogenated oils are man-made oils such as margarine. They are found in potato chips, most baked goods, candies, and most processed foods. Twinkies, lunch pies, and cookies tend to be made from hydrogenated fats. In addition, other junk foods such as french fries and potato chips are made from polyunsaturated fats such as sunflower oil, safflower oil, and corn oil. These fats lead to elevated amounts of inflammatory prostaglandins—potent hormones that trigger inflammation and raise cortisol levels. Unsaturated vegetable oils have been heat processed and are very unstable and nearly always turn rancid. Rancid oil causes oxidation in the body, which can lead to degenerative diseases because it may damage tissues. In addition, excessive amounts of these oils lead to an imbalance in female hormones.

Margarines are actually vegetable oils heated to very high temperatures under high pressure, which transforms them into unnatural hardened oils. A small amount of organic butter on occasion is much healthier than eating hydrogenated fats or heat-processed unsaturated vegetable oils. Cold-processed unsaturated vegetable oils found in health food stores are much healthier.

Avoid the fat substitute olestra, which is found in many snack foods such as potato chips. It can limit the absorption of carotenoids, which are rich yellow, orange, and red vegetables as well as dark green leafy vegetables, by as much as 50 percent.

Saturated fats

While you need a small amount of cholesterol, fatty meats and whole-milk products contain xenoestrogens, which can load your body up with even more estrogen and create huge hormonal imbalances. You can balance your consumption of saturated fats by avoiding fatty cuts of meat and limiting your amounts of dairy products such as butter, cheese, and whole milk.

Choose organic, fat-free varieties of milk, butter, and cheese, and choose organic eggs. Read the labels carefully. Many of these varieties have been produced free of hormones, but not all. In addition, free-range meats that have been raised to be free of synthetic hormones can also be purchased. Many grocery stores are now stocking these varieties. If you can't find them at your local grocery store, look for them at your favorite health food store, but always choose the leanest cuts. Instead of choosing red meat or pork, eat more fish, especially the fatty, cold-water fish such as salmon, mackerel, halibut, and tuna.

By avoiding animal fats, you will also avoid most oral intake of xenoestrogens, which (as stated in chapter 4) are chemicals that have estrogen-like activity. Xenoestrogens are found not only in plastics, but also in the hormones used by farmers and stockmen to fatten up their animals (turkeys, chickens, beef cattle, pigs, and hogs) for market.

Because of our continued exposure, xenoestrogens are slowly collecting in our tissues, especially the fatty tissues. This is probably the main reason we are witnessing such a major epidemic of premenopause symptoms in younger women and breast cancer in middle-aged and older women.

Here are some tips to help rid your body of xenoestrogens:

- Choose lean, free-range meats since the fat in regular meat is usually high in xenoestrogens.
- Choose organic foods because they are normally free of hormones and pesticides.
- Choose fat-free or low-fat dairy products.

Remember that phytoestrogens (the plant-based estrogen found in soybeans, for example) also block out estradiol and toxic xenoestrogens. Phytoestrogens will help your body decrease hot flashes, prevent osteoporosis, and assist your body in preventing vaginal dryness. In addition, diets that are high in phytoestrogens protect against breast and colon cancers.

Good fats

Just as hydrogenated fats are the most harmful fats (these are found in margarine, cakes, pies, cookies, and chips), there are also good fats that help to improve symptoms of PMS. These are:

- Black currant oil
- Borage oil
- Evening primrose oil

These oils contain high amounts of GLA, a very important fatty acid that stimulates the production of the good prostaglandins. They actually decrease inflammation, leading to a decrease in cortisol.

Extra-virgin olive oil is excellent for stir-frying and as a salad dressing. Good fats are also found in seeds and nuts, flaxseed oil, fish oils, and fatty fish such as salmon, mackerel, herring, halibut, and tuna. However, nuts go rancid easily; they should be kept in an airtight container and stored in the refrigerator or freezer.

Calories Do Count

Throughout this discussion of nutrition runs a theme of purposeful self-control, and that attention to wise choices should extend to the amount of food you eat as well. Calories do count, and the obesity epidemic is the clearest evidence of the fact.

Being overweight or obese significantly increases your risk of developing heart disease, diabetes, gallbladder disease, arthritis, and having a stroke and respiratory problems such as sleep apnea, as well as endometrial, breast, and colon cancers. Mortality rates increase significantly as BMI increases. In women particularly obesity is also associated with menstrual cycle irregularities, complications of pregnancy, male pattern hair growth, incontinence, and depression.

BMI

Body mass index, or BMI, is calculated by taking your weight (in pounds) and dividing it by your height squared (in inches), and then multiplying that by 703. Here is the mathematical formula:

$$BMI = \frac{W \text{ (lbs)}}{H \text{ (in)} \times H \text{ (in)}} \times 703$$

Look online for easy-to-use BMI calculators.

Nutritional Balance and Aging

As a woman ages, she has difficulty absorbing nutrients. This means that nutritional decisions must be made to help her balance her body during the aging process. When digestive enzymes aren't working at their optimal level, deficiencies occur.

This is especially true for B vitamins. To ensure that you make up the difference, you should eat plenty of leafy greens and whole grains. Adding brewer's yeast and wheat germ to your meals will further strengthen you against vitamin B depletion. Make sure that you consume enough fiber daily, such as oats, whole grains, raw vegetables, and ground flaxseeds. This will help to reduce toxins in your digestive tract and prevent constipation. Boost healthful bacteria in your digestive tract by eating yogurt and other fermented foods such as sauerkraut and kefir. These sources of healthy bacteria help to fight infections.

You can boost the antiaging powers of your next meal by adding fresh oregano. The USDA's agricultural research service tested the antioxidant action of twenty-one different fresh herbs, and found that all varieties of oregano came out on top, even ahead of vitamin E.

Besides eating citrus fruits, tomatoes, asparagus, and green leafy vegetables, take extra vitamin C every day to help fight free-radical damage, strengthen your immune system, and reduce your cancer risk. When you cook, add plenty of onion, garlic, or both to your dishes. Both have antioxidant and circulatory-boosting properties.

Make sure to consume quality protein daily at every meal. This will help to give you energy and provide your body with slow, even-burning fuel throughout the day. Sources include fish, lean chicken and turkey, and beans. Lower your risk of heart disease, cancer, and arthritis by eating foods rich in vitamin E and selenium, such as nuts, seeds, and vegetable oils.

As you age, dehydration becomes more of an issue. Make sure to stay well hydrated by drinking water every two hours whether you are thirsty or not, consuming half your body weight in ounces. Staying well hydrated can help cut your risk of chronic constipation, fatigue, headaches, weight gain, kidney malfunction, and poor absorption of nutrients. Pure water will keep you hydrated and help all of your body's systems to work more efficiently. In addition, water will help proper elimination, remove toxins, lessen arthritic pain, and help to transport proteins, vitamins, minerals, and sugars for assimilation. Water helps your body work at its best.

To ensure restful, recuperative sleep, eat complex carbohydrates, which can promote relaxation. Make sure to avoid caffeine, alcohol, or simple sugars in the evening as they will keep you awake or prevent a sound restorative sleep.

Begin now to practice caloric reduction. As you age, your body requires fewer calories; it also burns calories at a lower rate. In addition, a low-calorie diet has been shown to protect your DNA from damage. This will thereby prevent organ and tissue degeneration. Try to get more "bang for your caloric buck" by eating only high-quality, densely nutritious foods at each meal. Eat fresh fruits and vegetables, organically grown if possible.

God cares about what you eat, and He cares about the way you eat. That's why as your divine Creator He filled the earth with wonderfully delicious natural foods and other things to keep you healthy and satisfied. You may not live in the Garden of Eden, but many of the same nutritional choices that were provided there are still available to you. The Garden of Eden was a place of beauty and balance.

Chapter 15

VITAMINS AND SUPPLEMENTS
ESSENTIAL TO WOMEN'S HORMONE HEALTH

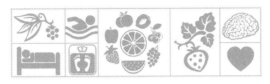

T HE DIVINE CREATOR richly supplied countless vitamins and minerals that He designed uniquely to help your body function at peak performance—including helping it maintain a delicate hormonal balance. Although vitamins and minerals are found in some measure in the foods we eat, taking supplemental vitamins and minerals will both restore your body to balance and keep it strong.

Women often overlook their nutritional requirements, becoming depleted and underinsured nutrient-wise. In addition, illness, age, and extreme diet practices may make it impossible to get all nutrients from food alone. For example, consuming enough calcium each day in the form of food and beverages is not realistic, so the simple solution is to take a calcium supplement.

What Is a Dietary Supplement?

Dietary supplements are intended to supplement the diet or increase total dietary intake and contain one or more of the following: vitamins, minerals, amino acids, herbs or other botanicals that can be concentrates, metabolites, constituents, extracts, or some combination of these. Not included in this definition but commonly found in supplements are animal-derived products and hormones. Within these categories, products may be pure single entities of known or unknown chemical components or mixtures in which all or none of the components may be known or unknown. The possible combinations boggle the mind. Consider the examples of dietary supplements in the following chart:

Dietary Supplement	Examples
Vitamins	B-complex (there are 12), such as vitamins B_1, B_2, niacin, or folic acid (water-soluble); vitamins A, D, E, and K (fat-soluble)

Dietary Supplement	Examples
Minerals	Calcium, magnesium, sodium, potassium, selenium, chromium, vanadium, copper, zinc
Herbs	Peppermint, chamomile, St. John's wort, kava, echinacea, goldenseal, ginseng, valerian, black cohosh, chasteberry (aka vitex), licorice, lavender
Enzymes	Pancreatic enzymes from animals or fruit such as pineapple and papaya (containing substances overset such as protease, lipase, amylase, etc.)
Animal-tissue-derived substances	Liver, adrenal, and thymus tissue from beef, pig, and sheep glands and organs
Nature-identical hormones and analogues	Progesterone cream synthesized from yams, estrogen concentrated from soy, dehydroepiandrosterone (DHEA) concentrated from yam
Natural metabolites	Antioxidants such as CoQ_{10}; phytonutrients such as flavonoids from citrus or pomegranate (ellagic acid); carotenoids (alpha and beta carotenes); policosanols from sugar cane
Mixtures	Products containing two or more ingredients from the same or assorted categories of dietary supplements: multivitamin mineral with or without an herbal base; traditional herbal formulations from India (Ayurvedic), China or Native North America; novel mixtures of herbs, vitamins, and enzymes.

Natural product chemists identify the molecules within foods and herbs that demonstrate potential to make a difference in how you feel and/or to change physiology and chemistry in your body, such as cholesterol or hormone levels. Supplements can selectively reinforce parts of the body that need more of a particular substance that might be difficult to get from the small amounts in food alone. When concentrated, they can enhance what is present in food or complement the diet by enhancing a food's potential to intentionally influence physical function.

What Are the Criteria for Safety and Efficacy?

The intention of a drug is to treat a health condition or relieve specific symptoms. The intention of a food is to nourish and support the body or improve its function, generally or specifically. The safety of both is tied to how much you can consume without side effects or risk of an adverse event. A special danger lies in combining dietary supplement products with over-the-counter or prescription medications. Ingredient safety is also directly associated with freedom from environmental pollutants, whether they come from the air, water, earth, unfriendly bacteria, or the manufacturing process.

How effective a product is—its efficacy—depends on preparation and dosage. Supplement companies are limited by law in what they can tell you about the actual health benefits of most natural products because that would make them sound like a drug—and they are licensed as a food product. A company is limited to structure and function statements with the recommended dose.

All dietary supplement manufacturers by law must adhere to good manufacturing practice (GMP) specifications just as rigorous as those affecting any food preparation manufacturer. The goal of the dietary supplement GMP regulations is to ensure that what is on the label is in the product every time a batch is manufactured, that there is no contamination, and that it disintegrates (to be appropriately absorbed) in thirty minutes after consumption.

It is not a valid criticism to say that the supplement industry is "unregulated." It is regulated. However, it is the choice of the company whether they wish to go further and adopt standards required for over-the-counter drugs or for pharmaceutical manufacturing. While there is no obligation for them to do so, there are dietary supplement companies and manufacturers who, in the spirit of excellence and concern over inferior and possibly injurious products, also voluntarily choose to do just that.

> *Note:* If you are pregnant, or plan on becoming pregnant, stop all supplements and consult your physician.

All botanical and supplemental products have a physiological action. If they didn't, there would be no point in taking them. Herbal products can alter normal body functions (and abnormal ones); therefore, it is important to understand and become informed consumers, sensitive to the possibility of herb/food/supplement and drug interactions, just as we should be with the potentially more life-threatening interactions between prescription drugs.

Concerns about possible interactions of herbs and drugs are especially warranted when an herb or combination of herbs has a focused effect similar to the intended drug. A synergy and antagonism between herb(s) and drug(s) may produce additive effects, amplifying the effect of the drug. For example, it could inhibit drug absorption, increase elimination, alter drug metabolism or excretion time, cause drug retention, or slow detoxification.

To protect yourself from adverse effects, follow these guidelines:

- Make sure you are honest about all the alternative approaches you are using by informing your prescribing physician and/or pharmacist.

- Take herbs and prescriptions at different times of the day.
- Be aware of plant allergies you have.
- Start with a low to moderate herb dose and work up.

Mind-Boggling, Isn't It?

Vitamins and minerals are important for bringing your body back into the right hormonal balance. But if you're like most people, looking at store shelves lined with bottles of vitamins and other supplements can leave you feeling a little mystified. If you do nothing more, at least take a good multivitamin/multimineral supplement daily.

Help balance the hormones in your body with zinc, vitamin B_6, all the other B-complex vitamins and 400 milligrams per day of magnesium. All of these can be found in a comprehensive multivitamin/multimineral supplement.

HOW MUCH IRON DOES A WOMAN NEED?[1]

Women who are menstruating or pregnant need more iron than postmenopausal women (or men). The amount of iron you need as a supplement depends on your diet. Vegetarians who do not eat meat, poultry, or seafood need almost twice as much iron as listed in the table because the body doesn't absorb nonheme iron in plant foods as well as heme iron in animal foods.

Life Stage	Recommended Amount
Teen girls (14–18)	15 mg
Adult women (19–50)	18 mg
Pregnant women	27 mg
Breastfeeding women	9 mg
Adult women (51 years and older)	8 mg

When choosing a multivitamin, look for "USP" on the label. This means that the product has been formulated to dissolve 75 percent after one hour in body fluids. For best absorption, take your multivitamin with meals and not on an empty stomach; otherwise you may experience nausea. Another important tip is to make sure that you take your multivitamin with a meal that contains a little fat. The fat-soluble vitamins A, D, and E need a little fat to get inside your system and go to work.

Select a multivitamin that includes a B-complex well in excess of the recommended daily dose. Ensure adequate amounts by not purchasing multivitamins you take once a day. They generally provide minimal amounts of supplements to prevent disease but do not augment organ and gland function or fortify reserves and strengthen the body's defenses. If you take this type of multivitamin, follow directions carefully; extra pills can result in too much vitamin A or D.

To improve tolerance, make sure that common allergens such as yeast, soy, milk, egg, wheat, corn, or artificial colorings are excluded. The label will give you dosage; a reputable company will keep within safe dosage. Avoid "mega-vitamins" that promise the moon but exceed safe limits and are less likely to have proper ratios between ingredients.

Beyond Multivitamins

Maybe you have heard someone say, "Taking vitamins results only in expensive urine." The truth is, all substances are eventually excreted, but as your vitamins go on their way through your bloodstream, they build your health and enhance your life. Keeping your body blanketed with the full spectrum of vitamins and minerals is likened to having an insurance policy that will help to ensure you against physical decline and degenerative disease. In 2002 the *Journal of the American Medical Association* reversed its twenty-year antivitamin stance, recommending that daily supplementation is a good thing.

Ultimately it is not what you take, it is what you absorb that counts; this is called bioavailability. You want your vitamin pill to break down within thirty minutes and mix with whatever food you are eating.

In addition to your multivitamin you will need to purchase a separate calcium supplement unless your multivitamin supplies a total of 1,000 milligrams in two or more doses per day. Do not waste your money on mega-doses. A midlife woman needs around 1,500 milligrams of calcium daily (800–1,000 milligrams before age fifty). The 1 percent of calcium not involved in building and strengthening bones and teeth ensures that your muscles contract correctly, that your blood will clot, and that nerves transport messages throughout your body. Depletion results in everything from insomnia and muscle cramps to agitation and depression, in addition to bone loss. If you do not consume enough calcium, your body will rob your bones to ensure it gets what it needs for these vital processes.

> Buy capsules of isoflavones or genistein at health food stores to help balance out your estrogen levels.

As is true of vitamins and minerals, food remains an important source of calcium, but many women cut out calcium-rich foods from their diets. This comes back to haunt them as they age, especially if they did not get adequate amounts during rapid bone-building time in their teens. Caffeine and soft drinks deplete calcium, as well as too much milk or sugar, excess fat, protein fiber, or alcohol. Medications such as tet-racycline, corticosteroids, antacids, sedatives, antibiotics, and muscle relaxants also deplete calcium. If you are "burpy" or gassy after meals, take calcium with breakfast; otherwise, calcium at night will help you sleep and reduce leg cramps.

PREMENOPAUSE SUPPLEMENTS

- Vitamin C: 1,000 milligrams daily
- Chromium: 200–400 micrograms daily (blood sugar balancer)
- Magnesium: 400–600 milligrams at bedtime
- Zinc: 15–30 milligrams daily
- Vanadyl sulfate: 5–10 milligrams daily (blood sugar balancer)
- Calcium: Bone and tooth builder
- Boron: 1–5 milligrams daily (maintenance of strong bones)
- Vitamin D: 100–400 international units daily (bone health)
- Vitamin E: 200–400 international units daily (antioxidant, protects the cardiovascular system)
- B complex: stress fighter

Use calcium carbonate when you need an antacid, but don't choose it as your best source of calcium. Calcium citrate is a better choice because it is well absorbed and slows bone loss. The "Cadillac" calcium is MCHC, or microcrystalline hydroxyapatite, a chemically complex raw bone concentrate. MCHC promotes bone remineralization in postmenopausal women. MCHC is a complete bone food containing naturally occurring calcium along with a spectrum of ultra-trace minerals embedded in biologically active protein, which contains all that is needed to build bone.

In addition to calcium supplementation, look also for a wide variety of antioxidants: natural-source carotenoids, lycopene, lutein, alpha carotene, cryptoxanthin, zeaxanthin and bioflavonoids such as quercetin and hesperidin. Many supplements are specific to the needs of either premenopausal or menopausal women, and further specific to the woman's personal symptoms.

For irregular periods the herb chasteberry, which is also called vitex, can help. This herb actually helps to stimulate the hypothalamus to increase the hormone LH. This, in turn, may help to stimulate the production of progesterone. Take 200 to 225 milligrams of a standardized extract of vitex a day or drink chasteberry tea.

> ## MIDLIFE SUPPLEMENTS
>
> - Flaxseed—helps keep the skin supple and vaginal tissues healthy; also helps the body produce prostaglandins (inflammation fighters)
> - Vitamin E—may reduce the risk of heart attack and stroke with 400 international units daily; is also a skin nutrient and mood balancer and relieves hot flashes. Check with your physician if you have hypertension, diabetes, or menstrual bleeding problems.
> - Fiber—keeps the body regular. Women who are constipated have four times the risk of breast cancer than women who are not.
> - Gamma oryzanol—derived from rice bran oil; a dose of 300 milligrams daily diminishes hot flashes, headaches, sleeplessness, and mood swings

Vitamin E can help to reduce breast tenderness. Take 400–800 international units daily. Purchase natural vitamin E, which is called d-alpha-tocopherol.

Gamma-linolenic acid (GLA) is an omega-6 fatty acid found in evening primrose oil, borage oil, and black currant oil. GLA may be helpful in controlling cyclic breast tenderness. The usual dose of GLA is 200–400 milligrams a day. Or you may take 4 grams of evening primrose oil a day or about 2 grams of borage oil a day. Be patient, however, for it may take a few months to notice the benefits of this.

Omega-3 fatty acids or EPA/DHA supplements you can trust

Increasing scientific evidence demonstrates that eicosapentaenoic acid (EPA) and docosahexaenoic acid (DHA), which your body does not make, powerfully influence cell membrane structure, composition, and function. They benefit skin along with cardiovascular, central nervous system, and retinal health. You must get them from food or supplements. An EPA/DHA supplement ensures proper hormone receptor function by either increasing or decreasing hormonal effects. If you supplement with "fish oil," quality is essential. The best choice for optimal absorption supplies EPA/DHA in triglyceride form. Buy from a company whose product is pharmaceutical grade and that guarantees it contains no harmful levels of mercury.

Other good sources of omega-3 come from flaxseed. Fresh ground organic flaxseed is preferred over the oil, but both are particularly helpful with hot flashes. The seeds provide both oil and flax fibers. The fibers are consumed by friendly bacteria in your colon and transformed into weak, but very beneficial, phytoSERMs (phyto = plant, SERM = selective estrogen receptor modulator). Should you wish to purchase flaxseed oil, the best way to use it is as a salad dressing.

IDENTIFYING ESSENTIAL OILS YOU CAN TRUST		
Essential Oils	Amount Per Serving (Range)	What You Should Know
Natural marine lipid concentrate, enteric-coated	1 gram	Look for supplements with enteric coating, which prevents repeating of fish oil taste and burping. If the label does not state the form of fish oil or guarantee freshness and purity, don't buy it.
EPA (eicosapentaenoic acid)	180–300 milligrams	
DHA (docosahexaenoic acid)	120–200 milligrams	Buying the concentrated oil is convenient and economical; 900 milligrams–1.5 grams of EPA daily.

Herbs

These time-tested and approved plants are truly gifts from God. He has given us every herb of the field for the healing and strengthening of our bodies. Many of our modern-day medicines are derived from herbs! Researchers all over the world know that herbs are very powerful and very effective. Research is ongoing as to how and why herbs can bring balance and healing to our lives. In Europe herbs have been used for centuries, and they continue to be used on a daily basis. Europeans have confidence in herbal therapy. Now Americans are embracing herbs as a way to prevent or to treat illness. However, education is key when it comes to taking herbs. They are powerful and must be treated with respect. Physicians are now seeing patients who are taking herbal remedies along with their prescribed medications. This can be very dangerous because there can be very real, very dangerous interactions, some life-threatening. Be sure to do your homework before you start using herbs to enhance your health.

Other supplements

It's not only about supplementing vitamins and minerals. A woman's body needs many other natural chemicals as she goes through life.

Ginseng. What benefits does ginseng provide? Ginseng is known as a plant-derived adaptogen, which simply means that it helps us "adapt" to the mental and physical rigors of our modern lifestyles. It is important to note that ginseng is the name given to three different plants. The most widely known is Panax ginseng, also known as Korean, Chinese, or Asian ginseng. Animal studies have shown that bioactive compounds in ginseng improve the sensitivity of the hypothalamic-pituitary-adrenal axis to cortisol. This axis also helps regulate your temperature, digestion, immune system, mood, sexuality, and energy usage and is a major part of the system that controls your reaction to stress, trauma, and injury. This means that ginseng provides protection against both physical and psychological stresses.

You can take 100–300 milligrams daily in the form of ginseng capsules, extract, or tea. Be sure not to mix ginseng with caffeine or another stimulant. The combination could cause palpitations.

Vitamins and minerals for depression. The following vitamins and minerals may be helpful in combating depression:

- Choline—this B-family vitamin may help push other B vitamins to the brain.
- Vitamin B_1—deficiency may lead to depression.
- Folic acid—low amounts of this member of the vitamin B family may be linked to depression.
- Vitamin B_2—proper levels may be linked to happiness.
- Vitamin B_3—deficiency may lead to worry, depression, and fear.
- Vitamin B_5—proper levels may lighten depression.
- Vitamin B_6—this B vitamin may help to quell emotional symptoms, especially in women. A link between vitamin B_6 deficiency and depression has been suggested.
- Vitamin B_{12}—deficiency may cause depression and confusion.
- Vitamin C—deficiency may lead to mental confusion and depression.
- Potassium—low levels may be associated with mood upsets, fatigue, and weakness, which are all symptoms of depression. Dietary sources of potassium include bananas, oranges, peas, and nonfat milk.
- Fish oil (omega-3 fatty acids)—researchers have suggested that fish oils may lessen the symptoms of depression as well as other midlife diseases, such as arthritis and heart disease.

Look for a good B-complex multivitamin that contains the full spectrum of B vitamins with folic acid and choline. This may help prevent deficiency.

If you are experiencing signs of depression, you should immediately avoid alcohol, caffeine, and sugar, all of which cause changes in energy and mood.

SAMe (S-Adenosyl-L-Methionine) is one of the safest and most effective antidepressants in the world. It works faster and more effectively than other antidepressants, with virtually no side effects.[2]

Its benefits include improved cognitive function and liver function, and a potential slowing of the aging process. As a matter of fact, some people take SAMe for its antiaging properties alone.

> ### SAMe—FOR DEPRESSION
>
> (Note: Refrigeration is recommended. Do not take with prescription antidepressants. For best results with SAMe, also take folic acid and vitamins B_{12} and B_6.)
> Form: capsule
> Dosage: 1,200–1,600 milligrams daily; take individual doses with food in the morning, midday, and late afternoon
> Frequency: three times daily, with meals

5-HTP is an intermediate in the natural synthesis of the essential amino acid tryptophan to serotonin. 5-HTP encourages brain serotonin levels that can lead to positive effects on emotional well-being.[3] Warning: do not use 5-HTP with prescription antidepressants.

Other supplements for depression

It has been theorized that the following supplements may have beneficial effects for depression and related mood disorders:

DHEA (dehydroepiandrosterone)—a hormone produced in the ovaries and glands of men and women. Though DHEA is important for good brain function, levels decline at midlife. DHEA relieves depression by improving psychological well-being. It may enhance memory, strengthen immunity, improve general physical condition, and make it easier to handle stress.[4]

Pregnenolone—a hormone produced by the ovaries and the adrenal glands. Depressed people have less than normal amounts of pregnenolone in their spinal fluid. It may increase the ability to handle stress, have a beneficial effect on the brain and nervous system, and improve the ability to retrieve and remember information.

Acetyl L-carnitine—an amino acid that has been reported to safely alleviate depression in some people. It may also possess cognitive-enhancing, antiaging effects. Dosage: 1,000 milligrams twice daily.

St. John's wort (hypericum)—an affordable herb that has been used for centuries to treat depression. This herb is used in Germany, where it is actually covered by health insurance. Noticeable results occur in about one month. Dosage: 300 milligrams three times daily. Please note that St. John's wort is not recommended for people who are taking MAO inhibitors. Note also that St. John's wort may interfere with other medications, including cancer medications. Consult your physician before using.

Depression, once identified, can be treated and overcome. Many people have developed their spiritual lives while walking through the dark valley of depression, emerging wiser and more grounded than ever before.

Supplements for a full life

Natural agents have the potential to help you age well with lots of energy and calm your moodiness, aches, and pains so you can function at a higher level. This is accomplished by supporting several organ and gland systems that directly and indirectly contribute to balanced hormone metabolism.

Ultimately a diet rich in a variety of fruits and vegetables, while limiting intake of animal protein and saturated fat, exercising until you sweat, honing coping skills, and committing to a fully expressed life are the keys to healthy aging and an uneventful menopause. Indeed, this is a mouthful, a "life-full"—and it is an achievable goal. Transformation comes about by enrolling in the process of self-examination and taking those baby steps. While you may never completely "arrive," you can get on the road. You may not be ready today, but this afternoon you might reconsider. How about tomorrow? So with this said, there are safe and effective interventions that hold the promise of helping you feel better quickly without mandating that you change every one of your eating and lifestyle habits.

WHAT VITAMINS AND MINERALS CAN DO		
Vitamins and Minerals With Established Recommended Daily Intakes (RDI)	Daily Amount/ Range	Desired Effect/Results
Fat-Soluble Vitamins		
Vitamin A (retinyl palmitate)	1,500–5,000 international units	Long-term use of vitamin A (>10,000 international units) may increase bone loss in an aging population. Carotenoids, containing beta carotene, are vitamin A precursors that can be ingested in unlimited amounts. The body converts beta carotene to vitamin A on an as-needed basis. Carotenoids also contribute health benefits as antioxidants in their unconverted form as immune protectors and for cancer prevention.

WHAT VITAMINS AND MINERALS CAN DO (Cont.)

Vitamins and Minerals With Established Recommended Daily Intakes (RDI)	Daily Amount/ Range	Desired Effect/Results
Beta carotene and/or natural carotenoids (measured as vitamin A equivalencies)	10,000–25,000 international units	
Vitamin D (as calciferol)	200–400 international units	As D_3 (cholecalciferol) aids calcium absorption. Conversion of vitamin D when exposed to sunlight most likely decreases with age.
Vitamin E (as d-alpha tocopheryl succinate or d-alpha tocopheryl acetate)	100–400 international units	Temporary boost to (3–6 months) 800–1200 IU for hot flash relief enhances immune system, relief of vaginal dryness, breast cysts and thyroid problems. Too much vitamin E can cause nausea, gas, or diarrhea. Large amounts (>800 international units) taken for a prolonged time period may increase bleeding time.
Water-Soluble Vitamins		
Vitamin C (as ascorbic acid)	200–1,200 milligrams	Builds collagen and maintains healthy gum, teeth, and blood vessels.
B-complex vitamins		Members of the B-complex vitamin family are water-soluble vitamins. They are washed away daily; they aid mood, mind, memory, and liver metabolism.
B_1 (as thiamine nitrate)	15–50 milligrams	Vitamin B_1 (thiamine) aids conversion of protein, carbohydrate, and fat into energy, detoxification, heart, and nervous systems. A shortage results in fatigue, depression, "pins and needles" sensations, or numbness in the legs.
B_2 (as riboflavin)	15–50 milligrams	Vitamin B_2 (riboflavin) aids cellular energy, hormone production, neurotransmitter function, healthy eyes and skin, and production of red blood cells.
B_3	50–500 milligrams	Niacin is important for release of energy from carbohydrates and the breakdown of fats and proteins. Niacin <10 milligrams per daily dose, otherwise can cause flushing. Niacinamide does not cause flushing, and it's beneficial for joint mobility.

WHAT VITAMINS AND MINERALS CAN DO (Cont.)		
Vitamins and Minerals With Established Recommended Daily Intakes (RDI)	Daily Amount/ Range	Desired Effect/Results
Pantothenic acid	100–500 milligrams	Improves cholesterol synthesis; participates in hormone synthesis
Water-Soluble Vitamins		
Vitamin B$_6$ (as pyridoxine hydrochloride)	20–100 milligrams	Vitamin B$_6$ (pyridoxine) is helpful in protein synthesis, manufacture of hormones, red blood cells, and over sixty enzymes and immune system function. Deficiency can result in a shortage of serotonin and contribute to depression.
Folate	200–800 micrograms	Folic acid/folate deficiency is credited in 30 percent of coronary heart disease, blood vessel disease, and strokes. Regulates cell division and supports healthy gums, red blood cells, gastrointestinal tract, immune system, and central nervous system. Alleviates depression in the elderly and protects against Alzheimer's.
Vitamin B$_{12}$	100–1,000 micrograms	Integral to a healthy nervous system; essential in the development of blood cells
Biotin	50–500 micrograms	Healthy hair and nails
Choline (as choline bitartrate)	50–500 milligrams	Improves fat metabolism
Inositol	50–500 milligrams	Inositol aids nerve transmission and fat metabolism and can help relieve depression
Para-amino benzoic acid (PABA)	10–50 milligrams	
Minerals		
Calcium	250–500 milligrams	Various forms absorbed to varying degrees

WHAT VITAMINS AND MINERALS CAN DO (Cont.)

Vitamins and Minerals With Established Recommended Daily Intakes (RDI)	Daily Amount/ Range	Desired Effect/Results
Magnesium (as any one or combination of glycinate, gluconate, citrate, or oxide)	250–500 milligrams	Magnesium in the form of citrate acts as a laxative above 400 milligrams a day. Magnesium oxide is poorly utilized when combined with calcium carbonate. If a multimineral formula or magnesium product uses the oxide or citrate forms, then be certain they are combined with other delivery systems, for example, a combination of glycinate, citrate, and oxide. Involved in over three hundred enzymatic reactions, including energy production. A deficiency intensifies reactions to stress by increasing the release of stress hormones.
Iron (as glycinate, citrate, or fumarate)	5–10 milligrams	Iron becomes less important after menopause and should not be taken in a supplement because it could increase heart risks.
Zinc (as aspartate, gluconate, citrate)	10–20 milligrams	All minerals are attached to carriers. The significance of carriers is controversial. Choose minerals attached to carriers that are known to absorb well and not affect stomach acid pH balance. Mineral carriers derived from vegetable protein, or individual amino acids are excellent.
Manganese (as aspartate, gluconate, glycinate)	1–2 milligrams	
Copper (as lysinate, amino acid chelate)	1–2 milligrams	
Avoid multivitamins/minerals with herbal bases or herb extracts. (They introduce the possibility of allergenicity and adulteration; their levels are generally too insignificant to be therapeutic.)		

Chapter 16

HEALTHY LIFESTYLE PRACTICES FOR EVERY WOMAN

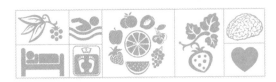

YOUR BODY IS in a dynamic state of hormonal flux every day, every hour, particularly as you grow older. This hormonal roller-coaster ride affects mood and behavior, temperature control, your skin, memory, and ability to sleep. It even affects the length of your life. Hormones are seriously influenced by the liver, adrenal and thyroid glands, and the ability of your body to maintain balanced blood sugar levels. This entire array of hormonal events and organ and glandular functions is influenced by select vitamins, minerals, botanicals, nonessential micronutrients, and more.

And yet no amount of nutrition, supplementation, exercise, and positive thinking will guarantee a lifetime of health. Health and hormonal balance may not be the ultimate goals anyway, but rather (important) components of the real life goal: happiness.

It comes down to *attitude*. Are you willing to expend some energy and time in order to be happy? Do you know how to achieve emotional balance?

BE AN OVERCOMER

What do you need to overcome in your attitude and outlook on life?

- Bitterness
- Negative thoughts
- Anxiety
- Sadness
- Excessive worry and stress
- Speaking destructive words instead of encouraging words
- Other: _____

Your attitude about life is significantly tied to your perception of your choices and the expectations to which you cling. No one has to repeat our family's medical or emotional heritage. We are free to educate ourselves, to choose to do it differently, to decide not to be around people or situations that diminish our emotional or physical well-being. When we choose to stay stuck, all we get for our effort is depression, anxiety, learned helplessness, and illness. A happy person takes steps to make changes. There is no waiting for the good life to drop from the sky. You will not feel better unless you decide to eat better. You cannot become physically fit by just thinking about it. You will not get organized by wishing you were. It takes work.[1]

There is evidence of a brain-immunity connection involving hormones influenced by a shift in more positive and hopeful attitudes. It has been said that faith has its own reward, but the fruit it bears is both spiritual and physical. Religiously active older people, those who go to services and participate in private religious activities, have lower blood pressure.[2] Research confirms that the faithful tend to lead longer lives.

Three-quarters of the studies about the healing power of prayer that were funded by the National Institutes of Health have demonstrated health benefits. Religion promotes fellowship, connection, and positive emotions. In general it is tied to a healthier lifestyle. There is little argument that prayer boosts morale, lowers agitation, loneliness, and life dissatisfaction, and enhances the ability to cope.[3]

Guilt Trips

What do you do with the feelings of guilt over your bad health being the product of your own choices and mishandled health remedies, the expectation that you must indeed have an ill-fated future? Do you berate yourself? "If only I had drunk all the milk Mother kept placing before me, I wouldn't be facing a decision about whether to take Fosamax....If only I had changed jobs instead of living under tyrannical pressure, maybe I could remember my daughter's phone number....If only I had walked around the block instead of sitting in the car drinking a latté while waiting for my ten-year-old to finish her piano lesson, I might not be twenty pounds overweight....If only...." Stop! Even if you had done all those things, there would still be a portion of every illness that remains out of your control. Despite "perfect" genetics and a rigorous health regimen, you may yet get breast cancer or Alzheimer's disease.

"Then why bother?" you ask. The answer is simple—the better your body is functioning, the greater chance you will have to be able to withstand serious and not-so-serious assaults to your health with energy and self-confidence. You may push back the onset of Alzheimer's to a point that you can remain at home to the end of your days without driving everyone crazy. You may die *with* breast cancer, not *from* it. And should none of those dire predictions come to pass, you will be blessed with more energy and vitality for life every day you live.

You are not a loser. You are not a failure. You are not guilty. You can do your best and make informed decisions—or not. Either way, you must hope and pray for the best. Accepting responsibility is important and can up the odds of feeling better, looking better, and living longer. Emotionally beating yourself up—feeling guilty—is sure to make you sicker.

Guilt can also make you fearful of trying to get well. The reasoning is, if you fail, you have proven you are a loser or there is no hope. The more nebulous the diagnoses of what is wrong with you, such as fibromyalgia, chronic fatigue, anxiety, and depression, the greater the tendency to blame yourself.

But the truth is, there is no one without a burden to bear. Granted, some are bigger than others. But if you feel that yours is the heaviest burden of all and that you are no longer surprised when a new problem gets added to the pile, your perspective may be off.

Looking for Blessings

Believing a lie can bring you into bondage and can cause you to passively accept circumstances or situations that you should never accept. For example, if you were told that you were created by God to be poor and broke, you might accept poverty. If your boss refused to pay you, you might accept that as your lot in life without even resisting. If thieves and robbers stole your goods, you might not even attempt to fight back. That acceptance would be created by the lie that caused you to allow poverty into your life in a way in which God never intended.

It works the same with your health. If you believe that the monthly discomfort of PMS is your lot in life as a woman, that belief system can then cause you to passively accept what God never intended rather than searching for a cure.

God has not cursed you. As a matter of fact, did you know that He has spoken great and powerful blessings over your life? Here are a few of them:

> And all these blessings will come on you and overtake you if you listen to the voice of the LORD your God.
>
> You will be blessed in the city and blessed in the field.
>
> Your offspring will be blessed, and the produce of your ground, and the offspring of your livestock, the increase of your herd and the flocks of your sheep.
>
> Your basket and your kneading bowl will be blessed.
>
> You will be blessed when you come in and blessed when you go out.
>
> The LORD will cause your enemies who rise up against you to be defeated before you; they will come out against you one way and flee before you seven ways.
>
> The LORD will command the blessing on you in your barns and in all that

you set your hand to do, and He will bless you in the land which the LORD your God is giving you.

—DEUTERONOMY 28:2–8, 11

Even in the face of all these powerful blessings, some might say, "Well, these blessings were for Israel, not for me." Not so! The Bible says, "Through Christ Jesus, God has blessed the Gentiles with the same blessing he promised to Abraham, so that we who are believers might receive the promised Holy Spirit through faith" (Gal. 3:14, NLT). "So don't worry about tomorrow, for tomorrow will bring its own worries. Today's trouble is enough for today" (Matt. 6:34, NLT). "You will keep in perfect peace all who trust in you, all whose thoughts are fixed on you!" (Isa. 26:3, NLT). "Give all your worries and cares to God, for he cares about you" (1 Pet. 5:7, NLT). Jesus said, "Come to Me, all you who labor and are heavily burdened, and I will give you rest" (Matt. 11:28). "If you know these things, blessed are you if you do them" (John 13:17).

Of course, when you're experiencing killer PMS or tragic infertility or monumental menopause symptoms, it might be difficult to think of your body as being especially blessed, but it is. With supernatural genius, God created your body as a living masterpiece—a divinely engineered work of art. And with just a little bit of God's wisdom, you can learn to work with your body to help it function better so that you will truly feel better.

Move It!

Our bodies were designed to move—to stretch, run, walk, jump, and play. You don't want to have trouble getting off the couch due to inactivity, stress, poor dietary habits, depression, fatigue, and lack of quality sleep.

We are living in an era when physical labor is not the norm. We live in a fast-paced, high-tech society where exercise must be a planned activity. Most of us do not farm land, milk cows, mow the back forty, or dig wells. We have reached an era of computerized washing machines, dishwashers, and robotic vacuum cleaners.

We are more advanced technically but more unhealthy physically than our grandmothers were. They experienced stress-relieving physical work that left them tired but satisfied at the end of each day. This differs from women today, who remain wired and tired day in and day out.

Exercise is a tonic with miraculous effects on mood, weight gain, energy levels, and sleep quality. In addition, exercise boosts immunity, is a natural appetite suppressant, improves HDL (the good cholesterol), creates pain-relieving endorphins, strengthens midlife bones, lowers the chance of cardiovascular disease, and improves circulation and respiration.

EXERCISE CHECKLIST

❏ Movement—I take every opportunity to increase my daily movement (walking instead of driving, taking the stairs instead of the elevator, etc.).

❏ Aerobic—I get thirty to sixty minutes of aerobic exercise, such as walking, running, swimming, cycling, etc., three to six days per week.

❏ Strength—I have a muscle workout routine that challenges me at least three times per week, such as weight lifting, core strengthening, etc.

❏ Stretching—I have a stretching routine I do at least three times per week.

❏ Support—I have an exercise partner or friend who encourages me and keeps me accountable, which in turn makes the activity more pleasurable.

If you persist in working hard without taking time for regular exercise, you will begin to notice, by midlife, that your back aches, your neck and shoulders are tight, your knees creak, and your hips hurt. Without regular exercise, you will become unable to deal with physical stress. It may be hard to believe, but the simple act of bending wrong or getting out of bed too fast can bring on a strained back or pulled muscles. The sooner you begin to nurture and care for your physical frame, the happier and healthier you will be.

The best prevention of functional decline with aging is based on continuing to be as physically and mentally active as possible while fueling your body with premium nutrition. There is no money to be made in pushing such a natural, simple solution. Nevertheless it remains the truth—and you know it. The "key" to aging well is already in your possession—embracing where you are, keeping out there, and monitoring your attitude.

Pathetically clinging to youth is a waste of energy in comparison to expending that energy by enriching one's life or maximizing the impact of a lifetime of experience by sharing it with that of younger generations.

Still, a few ways of hanging on to your youth do make sense. For example, some sources say that if you are a good veggie eater—five or more servings per day—you can consider yourself two years younger (and therefore two years less close to dying or becoming feeble) than you really are. You can take another year or more off your age by eating five ounces of nuts or three or more portions of fish weekly.

Your body does not require adoption of an extreme sport and hanging with twenty-year-olds to be in shape. Just taking Rover for his walk will pump additional blood to the brain, supply it with more oxygen and glucose, resulting in new capillaries and boosts in brain chemicals that are protective and strengthening of neurons and new neuronal connections. The Framingham Heart Study found that expending two thousand calories a week in physical activity (walking an hour per day) increased life expectancy by two years.[4]

SIMPLE WALKING PROGRAM

Don't look at walking as work. Instead, choose to see it as "your time," a special time for you to get away and enjoy the outdoors. Begin walking at a pace that is comfortable for you, briskly enough so that you cannot sing, but not so briskly that you cannot talk. Gradually increase your brisk walking time from thirty to sixty minutes, three or four times a week.

(NOTE: Each column indicates the number of minutes to walk. Complete three exercise sessions each week. If you find a particular week's pattern tiring, repeat it before going on to the next pattern. You do not have to complete the walking program in twelve weeks.)

Week	Walk	Walk Briskly	Walk	Minutes
1	5	5	5	15
2	5	7	5	17
3	5	9	5	19
4	5	11	5	21
5	5	13	5	23
6	5	15	5	25
7	5	18	5	28
8	5	20	5	30
9	5	23	5	33
10	5	26	5	36
11	5	28	5	38
12	5	30	5	40

Physical activity (only call it exercise if you want to) protects your heart by raising cardiac output, strengthening muscle, and improving blood supply, while benefiting almost every organ and system. It promotes increased intestinal motility, moving food along and decreasing inflammation, improving the function of the digestive system. Lower rates of cancer and diabetes, lowered blood pressure, and positive mood altering result from staying active—no pill will do as much.

You are a spiritual being who is having an earthly experience. Therefore, just as you nourish your body, you must feed your soul and nurture your spirit. The vicissitudes of life may lead you to self-examination and force you to take a deeper look at your life. Old, well-rooted beliefs may be unearthed and discarded. Or unbelief may be challenged or replaced with faith. Your spiritual health and personal faith in your Creator is the life-giving tonic that is hidden from the rest of the world. With daily cultivation and connection to God, you will experience the inner peace and ability to cope with life's challenges. Two strong beliefs will help you the most. First, you must have faith that God has a plan and purpose for your life. Second, you must have faith that He will work your trials out for your ultimate good, regardless of how your situation may look.

Fellowship with God equals true happiness. Many great people before us have confessed that without Him, life is meaningless. With Him, the possibilities are endless. Empires have been conquered and wars have been won when, to the natural mind, such outcomes seemed like impossibilities.

Spend time in prayer and meditation daily, live a life of service, and love unconditionally. By doing so you will add many meaningful years to your life.

Take the One-Year-to-Live Test

Pretend that you have only one year to live. What would you do during that time? Divide the things you would do into three categories:

- Things you enjoy doing
- Activities you must do
- Activities you neither enjoy nor have to do

Now eliminate all activities that you neither enjoy doing nor have to do. And for the remainder of your life, forget about them. Most women feel that they never get done in a day what should be done. If you eliminate the category three activities and focus only on the things that you enjoy doing and the things that you have to do, your stress level will decrease significantly and you will be much happier (quite likely healthier, as well).

Too often we try to carry our own burdens when the Lord wants to carry them for us. When we are led by the Lord, we can release the activities we should not be doing, and we can have the energy to do the things He desires for us to do. Reducing stress by giving Him your burdens will dramatically lessen the symptoms of premenopause or menopause.

What makes for a good attitude? While behavioral science journals are filled with what makes people emotionally sick, there is a dearth of research on what makes for happiness. What is known is that people who feel most content in life are most often married and have religious beliefs. Married people are happier than any other group; the religious more so than nonreligious. The thread that binds is a sense of connectedness. The basic truth is that we were made by our loving Creator for relationship. Our lives have increased meaning and purpose when we love and appreciate the value of others, ourselves and our God.

You do not have to be married to practice appreciation or love. You do have to involve your highest level of brain function to engage in loving activity. Love is a way of life—an outlook. Research indicates that appreciation is the purest, strongest form of love. It embraces optimism, courage, and some place to bestow our love. Such love is outward bound and strives for nothing for oneself. It is focused on family, friends, on our work or our passions. The capacity to love makes us brave and enables us to face all kinds of everyday situations. It is a great antidote to fear. And while we love, it heals, reducing stress, enhancing creativity, relieving pain, improving immunity, and reducing blood pressure.

....

Growing older: inevitable
Feeling older: optional

....

You will not develop an appreciative and loving spirit by focusing on all that is wrong. You must instead spend time building on your strengths and blessings. If this is hard for you, let this prayer be in your mind as you swing your feet out of bed, "Thank you for another day, and show me how I can be a blessing to someone." As you brush your teeth, give thanks for your blessings—your family, friends, the work or hobbies you enjoy, and the roof over your head.

If you cannot jog anymore, be thankful for the twenty years you were able to do such rigorous exercise, for the discipline it took and the contribution that it made to your current health. If you cannot eat some of the foods you loved in the past, be grateful for a body that knows better than you what is good for you. If hot flashes are waking you up, look on the time as "found time" in which you are blessed with uninterrupted time to pray. Do not waste time on your frailty or weaknesses. What do you continue to do well? How can you put your strengths to work to maximize your health or enrich life?

Contentment with life comes in recognizing we cannot always feel happy. If it were easy, we would not have to struggle so to find it. Happiness is realistic. It asks us to face the truth that our career ambitions and passions for worthy causes are worth fighting for, but not dying for. Our children remain a gift despite keeping us up nights wondering about their fate. Whether the pain of chemotherapy will improve quality or lengthen life remains unknown, but we march forward knowing we are doing our best for this moment in time.

Having the unrealistic expectation that every moment in life is supposed to be ecstatically joyful is a recipe for unhappiness. External efforts will never make it happen. Over 250,000 people die annually believing overindulgence and no exercise, along with the pleasure of food and drink, will bring happiness. The result is addiction, ill health, and death.

Happiness is like a visitor that comes and goes. Little things deliver it most consistently: receiving a call from a friend, having the energy to take a walk, hearing birds sing. Surely you have had the experience of achieving something that you were convinced would bring happiness, only to find grief instead. "If only I were healthy...rich...married...single...had lots of kids...lived in the country." Is your happiness dependent on an "if only"? Is an "if only" the source of pain? We live with our memories, disappointments, and illnesses. We can remain stuck in them or transcend them, using them to lift us to new understanding and wisdom.

Celebrate Life With a Merry Heart

Your life is meant to be a celebration—not a struggle! But too often whatever is happening (PMS symptoms, for example) can make you feel as if you are just barely getting by. Learn how to cultivate a merry heart—it will turn your entire outlook around. Having a merry heart is more powerful than any medicine to restore an exhausted, prematurely aging woman. The best medicine for overcoming stress and depression is laughter. In fact, the Bible says that "a merry heart does good like a medicine" (Prov. 17:22).

Norman Cousins wrote a book called *Anatomy of an Illness As Perceived by the Patient* in 1979. Cousins used laughter to fight a serious disease and actually laughed his way back to health. He watched funny movies and TV shows and read funny books. What he discovered has been proven true in the years since then. A good belly laugh is able to stimulate all the major organs like a massage. Laughter also helps to raise a person's energy level and helps to pull someone out of the pit of depression. Prescription for health: take laughter breaks every day. Find amusing things to watch and read. Laughter is contagious. Instead of looking critically at a difficult situation, find out what's funny about it. The average man or woman laughs only about four to eight times a day. The average child laughs about one hundred fifty times a day. Strengthen your immune system by becoming more childlike and laughing more often.

Quite plainly, joy gives you strength. The Bible says, "Don't be dejected and sad, for the joy of the LORD is your strength!" (Neh. 8:10, NLT). Circumstances don't matter, because it's truly possible to find joy, not in circumstances, but in Christ. And as Norm Cousins learned, joy leads to healing and sustained health.

Live in the Power of Forgiveness and Peace

It is critically important to forgive anyone who has wronged you. Ask the Holy Spirit to bring to your remembrance any unforgiveness that is hiding in your heart. Don't hold grudges, for they will eat away at your soul like a cancer. Jesus Christ did not sin or ever tell a lie. Although He was abused, He never tried to get even. And when He suffered, He made no threats. Instead, He had faith in God, who judges fairly. Since Jesus was punished for sin but didn't commit any, He was able to take your sin and everyone else's to the cross. He died so that you could be forgiven. Because of this great gift, you can find the power of forgiveness. If you have harbored hidden grudges and offenses against anyone—even God—right this moment give them to God. He will help you to walk in His own perfect peace.

Reject worry. Becoming anxious about your future will only serve to weaken you physically and spiritually. Worry never overcame anything, but joy overcomes everything:

> Rejoice in the Lord always. Again I will say, rejoice!…Be anxious for nothing, but in everything, by prayer and supplication with gratitude, make your requests known to God. And the peace of God, which surpasses all understanding, will protect your hearts and minds through Christ Jesus.
> —PHILIPPIANS 4:4–7

Replace worry with the confidence and peace that God has a wonderful plan for your whole life.

Break the power of negative words. Often women who are struggling with PMS and premenopause speak very negative words about their symptoms. You've probably heard them. They say things such as, "I've got the curse." Sadly such individuals don't realize that such words are powerful and can produce negative results. The Bible says, "The tongue can bring death or life; those who love to talk will reap the consequences" (Prov. 18:21, NLT). Take a moment once in a while to listen to your "self-talk." You might be surprised. If you are speaking negative words over yourself, stop. Ask God to fill your mouth with genuine appreciation and gratitude for everything in your life, including the precious gift of procreation and all the hormonal events that come with it.

Have you experienced concerns over your hormonally induced symptoms? Have you had doubts about yourself when you felt out of sorts? Rest assured that nothing about your life has gone out of control. God is gracing your life with a wonderful season of change. This special time of change is from Him. Embrace your new season with grace, excitement, and peace through the power of faith.

Overcome your stress with faith. Many American women are entering premenopause and menopause at an early age, in part because of the tremendous stress of their lifestyles. The hormonal balance of estrogen and progesterone, as well as deficiencies of these hormones, relates to the amount of stress that is faced daily. To overcome your stress, try simple spiritual steps:

Fix your attention on God—not on your problems. Dwelling on your problems produces inner turmoil and blocks the power of Christ, the Prince of Peace, from comforting and calming you.

Pray and thank God for all of His blessings. When stressed, you may tend to forget all that God has done and is doing in your life. Yet your blessings far outweigh any temporary crisis. As you pray for your needs, also thank God for His providential care.

Eliminate negative thoughts by meditating on uplifting thoughts. You become what you think (Prov. 23:7). Therefore, instead of dwelling on what stresses you, clean out negative thoughts, replacing them with the joy-filled attitudes described in the Bible.

Pray. Prayer is a limitless resource for filling your life with God's Spirit, wisdom, and strength. He will strengthen your body and give you the determination to take the natural steps you need to take in order to walk in health. The Bible says, "You shall know the truth, and the truth shall set you free" (John 8:32). Now you may never have considered that this scripture included hormonal problems, but it does. It concerns all truth—even the truth about your body and your health!

You can rise above the discomforts of your particular set of physical, mental, and emotional challenges. Through the power of good nutrition, healthy lifestyle choices, exercise, vitamins, and supplements, and most importantly of all, through the power of dynamic faith, you can be empowered to halt the decline and turn your life around.

With God's grace, mental acuity, physical strength, and increasing joy await you.

Healthy living is not an exercise in deprivation. Once you get on the path, it is self-motivating.

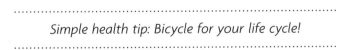

Simple health tip: Bicycle for your life cycle!

Today there is no excuse to not be educated about every aspect of your health. Education gives hope and knowledge to do better. The more you know, the more discerning you can be. There is, indeed, a lot of pressure to ignore one's reality, to hurry or to cut corners. But being healthy requires you to set reasonable goals—that you build on small steps while focusing on what life will look like when you get past thinking that you have to have that doughnut or clean your plate. What will it take to make it important enough to change your ways or will you wait for the crisis?

A-B-C FOR LIFE

A—Antiaging antioxidant: Vitamin E is an antiaging antioxidant that reduces the risk of heart attack by acting as an anticoagulant and vasodilator against blood clots and retards cellular and mental aging.
B—Breathe well. Proper breathing will help you relax. Start from the very bottom of your lungs and breathe in slowly through your nose.
C—Commit to continued improvement in all areas of your hormonal health.

The bottom line is: you are competent and powerful; you have choices. Let others know what you need and do not need from them. "'Fess up" should you require help in overcoming blocks to getting started. It is never too late to do the right thing.

Women face very real hormone issues, and our faith in the medical profession and technology has been shaken. But we still have an abundance of physical information upon which we can exercise our critical thinking skills, and we have spiritual and emotional mentors who can show us the best way to go. Not only can you find your personal optimal wellness, but you also may be able to influence and nurture those with whom you come into contact.

By applying faith to every curve and bump along the way, you can make it through every transition with grace and peace and enter into the wonderful things that God has waiting for you around the corner. Keep learning, and keep looking to Him for guidance. This next season in your life will be the best one yet. With faith in God, you cannot fail!

NOTES

Chapter 1
We're All Women Here

1. C. J. Gruber et al., "Mechanisms of Disease: Production and Actions of Estrogens," *NEJM* 346(5) (2002): 340–352.

Chapter 2
When Things Are Out of Balance

1. MedlinePlus, "Hormones," http://www.nlm.nih.gov/medlineplus/hormones.html (accessed January 14, 2015).

2. SEER Training Modules, "Endocrine Glands and Their Hormones," National Cancer Institute, http://training.seer.cancer.gov/anatomy/endocrine/glands/ (accessed January 15, 2015).

3. CDC, "Prevalence of Disabilities and Associated Health Conditions Among Adults—United States (1999)," *Morbidity and Mortality Weekly Report* 50 (2001): 120–125.

4. Sylvia Wassertheil-Smoller et al., "Effect of Estrogen Plus Progestin on Stroke in Postmenopausal Women: The Woman's Health Initiative: A Randomized Trial," *Journal of the American Medical Association* 289 (May 28, 2003): 2673–2684.

Chapter 3
They Meant Well

1. C. P. L. de Gardanne, *De la Menopause ou de l'Âge Critique des Femmes* (Paris: Chez Mequignon, Marvis, Libraire, 1821).

2. A. M. Farnham, "Alienist," *Neurologist* 8, no. 582 (1887).

3. Ibid.

4. Suzanne W. Fletcher and Graham A. Colditz, "Failure of Estrogen Plus Progestin Therapy for Prevention," *Journal of the American Medical Association* 288, no. 3 (2002): 366–368.

5. Grady D. Herrington et al., "Cardiovascular Disease Outcomes During 6–8 Years of Hormone Therapy," Heart and Estrogen/Progestin Replacement Study Follow-Up (HERS II), *Journal of the American Medical Association* 288 (2002): 49–57.

6. K. Johnson, "HRT Linked to Increase in Urinary Incontinence," *OBGyn News* 38, no. 12 (June 15, 2003): 1–2.

7. Writing Group for the Women's Health Initiative Investigation, "Risks and Benefits of Estrogen Plus Progestin in Healthy Menopausal Women: Principal Results From the Women's Health Initiative Randomized Controlled Trial," *Journal of the American Medical Association* 28 (2002): 321–333.

8. Adapted from "Writing Group for the Women's Health Initiative Investigation," *Journal of the American Medical Association* 288 (2002): 321.

9. W. F. Posthuma et al., "Cardioprotective Effect of Hormone Replacement Therapy in Postmenopausal Women: Is the Evidence Biased?," *British Medical Journal* 308, no. 6939 (1994): 1268–9.

Chapter 4
Regulating PMS Symptoms and Menstrual Cycles

1. WomensHealth.gov, "Infertility," http://www.womenshealth.gov/publications/our-publications/
   fact-sheet/infertility.pdf (accessed January 16, 2015).

2. M. Yusoff Dawood, "Primary Dysmenorrhea: Advances in Pathogenesis and Management,"
   Obstetrics and Gynecology 108 (August 2006): 428–441.

3. A. F. Walker et al., "Magnesium Supplementation Alleviates Premenstrual Symptoms of Fluid
   Retention." *Journal of Women's Health* 7, no. 9 (1998): 1157–1165.

4. James LaValle, "Guide to Herb, Vitamin, and Mineral Use," *OB/GYN Special Edition*, Spring
   1999.

5. R. L. Reid and S. S. C. Yen, "Premenstrual Syndrome," *American Journal of Obstetrics and
   Gynecology* 139 (1981): 85–104.

6. American Association of Clinical Endocrinologists, "Position Statement on Metabolic and Cardiovascular Consequences of Polycystic Ovary Syndrome," *Endocrine Practice* 11, no. 2 (2005):
   126–134.

Chapter 5
Premenopause, Menopause, Postmenopause

1. R. D. Gambrell, R. C. Maier, and B. I. Sanders, "Decreased Incidence of Breast Cancer in Post-
   menopausal Estrogen-Progesterone Users," *Obstetrics and Gynecology* 62 (1983): 435–443;
   John R. Lee, "Osteoporosis Reversal: The Role of Progesterone," *International Clinical Nutri-
   tion* Review 10, no. 3 (July 1990): 384–391; O. Picazo and A. Fernandez-Guasti, "Anti-Anxiety
   Effects of Progesterone and Some of Its Reduced Metabolites: An Evaluation Using the Burying
   Behavior Test," *Brain Research* 680 (May 1995): 135–141; J. C. Prior, "Progesterone as a Bone
   Trophic Hormone," *Endocrine Reviews* 11, no. 2 (May 1990): 386–398.

2. John R. Lee, Jesse Hanley, and Virginia Hopkins, *What Your Doctor May Not Tell You About
   Premenopause* (New York: Warner Books, 1999), 60.

3. L. Dennerstein et al., "A Prospective Population-Based Study of Menopausal Symptoms,"
   Obstetrics and Gynecology 96 (2000): 351–358.

4. C. M. Hasler, "The Cardiovascular Effects of Soy Products," *Journal of Cardiovascular Nursing*
   16, no. 4 (July 2002): 50–63; M. J. Messina, "Soy Foods and Soybean Isoflavones and Menopausal Health," *Nutrition in Clinical Care* 5, no. 6 (November–December 2002): 272–282; L.
   W. Lissin and J. P. Cooke, "Phytoestrogens and Coronary Heart Disease," *Journal of American
   College of Cardiology* 35, no. 6 (May 2000): 1403–1410; T. B. Clarkson and M. S. Anthony,
   "Phyoestrogens and Coronary Heart Disease," *Baillieres Clinical Endocrinology and Metabolism* 12, no. 4 (December 1998): 589–604; G. Burke et al., "Soy Protein and Isoflavone Effects
   on Vasomotor Symptoms in Peri- and Postmenopausal Women: The Soy Estrogen Alternative
   Study," *Menopause* 10, no. 2 (2003): 147–153.

5. Kate Murphy, "The Dark Side of Soy," BusinessWeek.com, December 18, 2000, http://www
   .businessweek.com/2000/00_51/b3712218.htm (accessed March 2, 2015).

6. E. Liske, "Therapeutic Efficacy and Safety of *Cimicifuga Racemosa* for Gynecologic Disorders,"
   Advances in Therapy 15 (1998): 45–53.

7. S. Lieberman, "A Review of the Effectiveness of *Cimicifuga Racemosa* (Black Cohosh) for the
   Symptoms of Menopause," *Journal of Women's Health* 7, no. 5 (June 1998): 525–529; A. Petho,
   "Menopausal Complaints: Changeover of a Hormone Treatment to an Herbal Gynecological
   Remedy Practicable?" *Ärztliche Praxis Gynäkol* 38 (1987): 1551–1553.

8. V. Stearns et al., "A Pilot Trial Assessing the Efficacy of Paroxetine Hydrochloride (Paxil) in Controlling Hot Flashes in Breast Cancer Survivors," *Annals of Oncology* 11 (2000): 17–22.

9. J. Trabal, "Hormonal Changes Associated With Menopause," *Therapeutic Interventions in Menopause: The Role of Estrogens* (August 2000): 4.

10. L. Boothby et al., "Bio-Identical Hormone Therapy: A Review," *Menopause* 11, no. 3 (2004): 356–365.

11. National Institutes of Health, "Questions and Answers About Estrogen-Plus-Progestin Hormone Therapy."

Chapter 6
Mood Swings—Stress, Anger, Depression, and Anxiety

1. S. E. Taylor et al., "Female Responses to Stress: Tend and Befriend, Not Fight or Flight," *Psychological Review* 107, no. 3 (2000): 419–429.

Chapter 7
Heart Disease

1. CardioSmart, "Heart Disease Statistics," American College of Cardiology, https://www.cardiosmart.org/Heart-Basics/CVD-Stats(accessed March 2, 2015).

2. K. J. Mukamal et al., "Tea Consumption and Mortality Rates After Acute Myocardial Infarction," *Circulation* 105(21) (May 28 2002): 2476–81; J. D. Lambert and C. S. Yang, "Cancer Chemopreventative Activity and Bioavailability of Tea and Tea Polyphenols," *Mutation Research* 523–524 (February–March 2003): 201–208.

3. American Heart Association, "Statistical Fact Sheet—2014 Update, Women and Cardiovascular Diseases," http://www.heart.org/idc/groups/heart-public/@wcm/@sop/@smd/documents/downloadable/ucm_462030.pdf (accessed January 19, 2015).

4. Frank B. Hu and W. C. Willett, "Optimal Diets for Prevention of Coronary Heart Disease," *Journal of the American Medical Association* 288, no. 20 (2002): 2569–2578.

5. E. Guallar and Inmaculada Sanz-Gallardo, "Mercury, Fish Oils, and the Risk of Myocardial Infarction," *New England Journal of Medicine* 347, no. 22 (2002): 1747–1754.

6. W. E. Kraus and J. A. Houmard, "Effects of the Amount and Intensity of Exercise on Plasma Lipoproteins," *New England Journal of Medicine* 347, no. 19 (2002): 1483–1492.

7. T. Zheng et al., "Glutathione 2-transferase M1 and T1 Genetic Polymorphisms, Alcohol Consumption and Breast Cancer Risk," *British Journal of Cancer* 88, no. 1 (January 13, 2003): 58–62.

8. To calculate BMI, see, for example, http://www.webmd.com/diet/body-bmi-calculator.

9. FamilyDoctor.org, "High Blood Pressure: Diagnosis & Tests," August, 2014 http://familydoctor.org/familydoctor/en/diseases-conditions/high-blood-pressure/diagnosis-tests.html (accessed January 19, 2015).

10. M. R. Joffres, D. M. Reed and K. Yano, "Relationship of Magnesium Intake and Other Dietary Factors to Blood Pressure: the Honolulu Heart Study," *American Journal of Clinical Nutrition* 45(2) (February 1987): 469–476.

11. N. M. Rao et al., "Angiotensin Converting Enzyme Inhibitors From Ripened and Unripened Bananas," *Current Science* 76 (1999): 86–88.

Chapter 8
Breast and Other Women's Cancers

1. National Cancer Institute, "Breast Cancer," http://www.cancer.gov/cancertopics/types/breast (accessed January 19, 2015).

2. American Cancer Society, "What Are the Key Statistics About Breast Cancer?" http://www .cancer.org/cancer/breastcancer/detailedguide/breast-cancer-key-statistics (accessed January 19, 2015).

3. American Cancer Society, "Breast Cancer: Facts and Figures 2013–2014," http://www.cancer .org/acs/groups/content/@research/documents/document/acspc-042725.pdf (accessed January 19, 2015).

4. American Cancer Society, "What Are the Key Statistics About Breast Cancer?"

5. Health Canada, "It's Your Health: Breast Cancer," http://publications.gc.ca/collections/ collection_2008/hc-sc/H50-3-157-2004E.pdf (accessed January 19, 2015).

6. D. D. Baird et al., "Dietary Intervention Study to Assess Estrogenicity of Dietary Soy Among Postmenopausal Women," *Journal of Clinical Endocrinology and Metabolism* 80 (1995): 1685–1690.

7. M. Messina et al., "Gaining Insight Into the Health Effects of Soy but a Long Way Still to Go: Commentary on the Fourth International Symposium on the Role of Soy in Preventing and Treating Chronic Disease," *Journal of Nutrition* 132 (2002): 547S–551S.

8. R. K. Tiwari et al., "Selective Responsiveness of Human Breast Cancer Cells to Indole-3-Carbinol, a Chemopreventive Agent," *Journal of the National Cancer Institute* 86, no. 2 (January 1994): 126–131.

9. L. Nystrom et al., "Long-Term Effects of Mammography Screening: Updated Overview of the Swedish Randomised Trials," *Lancet* 359 (March 16, 2002): 909–919.

10. American Cancer Society, "What Are the Key Statistics About Cervical Cancer?" July 19, 2014, http://www.cancer.org/cancer/cervicalcancer/detailedguide/cervical-cancer-key-statistics (accessed January 19, 2015).

11. Ibid.

12. University of Texas, MD Anderson Cancer Center, "Uterine Cancer Research Program," http:// www.mdanderson.org/education-and-research/research-at-md-anderson/basic-science/research -programs/uterine-cancer-research-program/index.html (accessed January 19, 2015).

13. University of Texas, MD Anderson Cancer Center, "Uterine Cancer Prevention and Screening," http://www.mdanderson.org/patient-and-cancer-information/cancer-information/cancer-types/ uterine-cancer/prevention/index.html (accessed January 19, 2015).

14. National Cancer Institute, "Ovarian Cancer," http://www.cancer.gov/cancertopics/types/ovarian (accessed January 19, 2015).

15. National Cancer Institute, "General Information about Ovarian Epithelial Cancer," http://www .cancer.gov/cancertopics/pdq/treatment/ovarianepithelial/Patient (accessed January 19, 2015).

16. American Cancer Society, "Survival Rates for Ovarian Cancer, by Stage," http://www.cancer.org/ cancer/ovariancancer/detailedguide/ovarian-cancer-survival-rates (accessed January 19, 2015).

17. L. S. Cook, M. L. Kamb, and N. S. Weiss, "Perineal Powder Exposure and the Risk of Ovarian Cancer," *American Journal of Epidemiology* 145, no. 5 (March 1997): 459–465.

Chapter 9
Osteoporosis

1. Tori Hudson, *Women's Encyclopedia of Natural Medicine* (New York: McGraw Hill Companies, 2008), 238.

2. William S. Pietrzak, *Musculoskeletal Tissue Regeneration* (New York: Humana Press, 2008), 48.

3. Hudson, *Women's Encyclopedia of Natural Medicine*.

4. Pietrzak, *Musculoskeletal Tissue Regeneration*.

5. HealthyNewAge.com, "Osteoporosis Home Test," http://www.healthynewage.com/osteoporosis-progesterone.htm (accessed January 20, 2015).

6. Ernesto Canalis, Andrea Giustina, and John P. Bilezikian, "Mechanisms of Anabolic Therapies for Osteoporosis," *New England Journal of Medicine* 357, no. 9 (August 30, 2007): 905–916.

7. Adapted from Carolyn Riester O'Connor and Sharon Perkins, *Osteoporosis for Dummies* (Indianapolis, IN: Wiley Publishing Inc., 2005), 134–135.

8. *Obstetrics and Gynecology* 104, "Hormone Therapy: Osteoporosis" (2004): S66–S76.

9. National Institute of Arthritis and Musculoskeletal and Skin Disorders, "Information About the Musculoskeletal and Skin Systems," http://science.education.nih.gov/supplements/nih6/Bone/guide/info_musculo_skin-a.htm (accessed January 20, 2015).

10. Herbal-Supplements-Guide.com, "Best Calcium Supplements," http://www.herbal-supplements-guide.com/best-calcium-supplements.html (accessed January 20, 2015).

11. Jack Challem, ed., *User's Guide to Nutritional Supplements* (North Bergen, NJ: Basic Health Publications Inc., 2003).

12. Brigham and Women's Hospital, "Hip Fracture," http://healthlibrary.brighamandwomens.org/Library/Encyclopedia/85,P08957 (accessed January 20, 2015).

13. UW Medicine Department of Radiology, "Osteopenia," http://www.rad.washington.edu/academics/academic-sections/msk/teaching-materials/online-musculoskeletal-radiology-book/osteopenia (accessed January 20, 2015).

14. World Health Organization, "Who Scientific Group on the Assessment of Osteoporosis at Primary Health Care Level," http://www.who.int/chp/topics/Osteoporosis.pdf (accessed January 20, 2015).

15. D. Cerimele, L. Celleno, and F. Serri, "Physiological Changes in Ageing Skin," *British Journal of Dermatology* 122, no. 35 (April 1990): S13–S20.

16. National Institutes of Health, "Calcium Fact Sheet for Consumers," http://ods.od.nih.gov/factsheets/Calcium-Consumer/ (accessed January 20, 2015).

17. AlgaeCal.com, "Calcium Absorption—Bioavailability and Solubility," http://www.algaecal.com/calcium-absorption.html (accessed January 20, 2015).

18. National Cancer Institute, "Calcium and Cancer Prevention: Strengths and Limits of the Evidence," http://www.cancer.gov/cancertopics/factsheet/prevention/calcium (accessed January 20, 2015).

Chapter 10
Weight Management

1. Or use an online BMI calculator such as http://www.webmd.com/diet/body-bmi-calculator.

2. A. H. Mokdad et al., "Prevalence of Obesity, Diabetes, and Obesity Related Health Risk Factors, 2001," *Journal of the American Medical Association* 289, no. 1 (2003): 76–79.

3. Edward R. Rosick, "Cortisol, Stress, and Health," *Life Extension,* December 2005 http://www.lef
.org/magazine/2005/12/report_cortisol/Page-02 (accessed January 20, 2015).

4. Centers for Disease Control and Prevention, "Physical Activity: Why Strength Training?"
http://www.cdc.gov/physicalactivity/growingstronger/why/index.html (accessed January 20,
2015).

5. Georgia State University, "Strength Training Main Page," Department of Kinesiology and
Health, http://www2.gsu.edu/~wwwfit/strength.html (accessed January 20, 2015).

Chapter 11
Memory and Mental Clarity

1. Adapted from Dharma Khalsa, *Brain Longevity* (New York: Warner Books, Inc., 1997).

2. W. D. Heiss et al., "Activation of PET as an Instrument to Determine Therapeutic Efficacy in
Alzheimer's Disease," *Annals of the New York Academy of Sciences* 695 (1993): 327–331.

3. Suvi Rovio, Ingemar Kareholt, and Eeva-Liisa Helkala, "Leisure-time Physical Activity at
Midlife and the Risk of Dementia and Alzheimer's Disease," *The Lancet Neurology* 4, no. 11
(November 2005): 705–711; Eric Larson et al., "Exercise Is Associated With Reduced Risk for
Incident Dementia Among Persons Sixty-Five Years of Age and Older," *Annals of Internal
Medicine* 144, no. 2 (January 17, 2006): 73–81.

4. William T. Greenough, Neal J. Cohen, and Janice M. Juraska, "New Neurons in Old Brains:
Learning to Survive?" *Nature Neuroscience* 2 (1999), 203–205.

5. Cenacchi et al., "Cognitive Decline in the Elderly: A Double-Blind, Placebo-Controlled Multi-
center Study on Efficacy of Phosphatidylserine Administration," *Aging* (Milano) 5, no. 2 (April
1993): 123–33.

Chapter 12
Sleeplessness and Insomnia

1. National Sleep Foundation, "Women and Sleep," http://sleepfoundation.org/sleep-topics/women
-and-sleep (accessed January 20, 2015).

2. Better Health Channel, "Sleep Deprivation," http://www.betterhealth.vic.gov.au/bhcv2/
bhcarticles.nsf/pages/Sleep_deprivation?OpenDocument (accessed January 20, 2015).

3. College of Nursing Villanova University, "Symptoms of Sleep Deprivation," http://nurseweb
.villanova.edu/womenwithdisabilities/sleep/slpdep.htm (accessed January 20, 2015).

4. M. W. Johns, "A New Method for Measuring Daytime Sleepiness: The Epworth Sleepiness
Scale," *Sleep* 14 (1991): 540–545. Copyright M. W. Johns, 1990–1997. Reproduced with permis-
sion.

5. J. R. Thomas et al., "Tyrosine Improves Working Memory in a Multitasking Environment,"
Pharmacology, Biochemistry, and Behavior 64, no. 3 (November 1999): 495–500.

6. E. U. Vorbach et al., "Therapy for Insomnia: Efficacy and Tolerability of a Valerian Preparation.
600 mg of Valerian," *Psychopharmakotherapie* 3 (1996): 109–115.

7. Sally Squires, "Back to Basics," *Washington Post,* September 25, 2001, F1.

Chapter 13
Fight Aging by Restoring Hormone Balance

1. As quoted in Christiane Northrup, *Women's Bodies, Women's Wisdom* (New York: Bantam
Books, 2010), 754. Viewed at Google Books.

2. Thinkexist.com, "Carl Bard Quotes," http://thinkexist.com/quotes/carl_bard/ (accessed January 20, 2015).

Chapter 14
Foods Essential to Women's Hormone Health

1. S. J. Baek et al., "Resveratrol Enhances the Expression of Nonsteroidal Anti-inflammatory Drug-Activated Gene (NAG1) by Increasing the Expression of p53," *Carcinogenesis* 23(3) (2002): 425–343.

2. E. T. Eng et al., "Anti-aromatase Chemicals in Red Wine," *Annals of the New York Academy of Sciences* 963 (2002): 239–246.

3. 34 Menopause Symptoms, "Fewer Japanese Women Experience Night Sweats," http://www.34-menopause-symptoms.com/fewer-japanese-women-experience-night-sweats.htm (accessed January 20, 2015).

4. María I. Gil et al., "Antioxidant Activity of Pomegranate Juice and Its Relationship With Phenolic Composition and Processing," *Journal of Agricultural and Food Chemistry* 48, no. 10 (2000): 4581–4589.

5. Salahuddin Ahmed et al., "*Punica Granatum L.* Extract Inhibits IL-1ß Induced Expression of Matrix Metalloproteinases by Inhibiting the Activation of MAP Kinases and NF-B in Human Chondrocytes In Vitro," *Journal of Nutrition* 135 (2005): 2096–2102.

6. H. M. Kwak et al., "Beta- Secretase (BACE1) Inhibitors From Pomegranate Husk," *Archives Pharmacal Research* 28 (2005): 1328–1332.

7. Linda Page, *Healthy Healing*, 11th ed. (N.p.: Traditional Wisdom Inc., 2000), 170.

Chapter 15
Vitamins and Supplements Essential to Women's Hormone Health

1. From "Iron: Fact Sheet," National Institutes of Health, http://ods.od.nih.gov/factsheets/Iron-Consumer/ (accessed November 11, 2014).

2. J. F. Rosenbaum et al., "The Antidepressant Potential of Oral S-Adenosyl-L-Methionine," *Acta Psychiatrica Scandinavica* 81, no. 5 (May 1990): 432–436.

3. K. Zmilacher et al., "L-5- Hydroxytryptophan Alone and in Combination With a Peripheral Decarboxylase Inhibitor in the Treatment of Depression," *Neuropsychobiology* 20, no. 1 (1988): 28–35.

4. O. M. Wolkowitz, "Antidepressant and Cognition-Enhancing Effects of DHEA in Major Depression," *Annals of the New York Academy of Sciences* 774 (December 1995): 337–339.

Chapter 16
Healthy Lifestyle Practices for Every Woman

1. D. Baker and C. Stauth, *What Happy People Know: How the New Science of Happiness Can Change Your Life for the Better* (Emmaus, PA: Rodale, 2002).

2. H. G. Koenig, "The Relationship Between Religious Activities and Blood Pressure in Older Adults," *International Journal of Psychiatry in Medicine* 28, no. 2 (1998): 159–263.

3. D. Hales, "Why Prayer Could Be Good Medicine," *Parade* (March 23, 2003): 4–5.

4. M. W. D'Agostino et al., "Primary and Subsequent Coronary Risk Appraisal: New Results From the Framingham Study," *American Heart Journal* 139 (2000):272–281.

INDEX

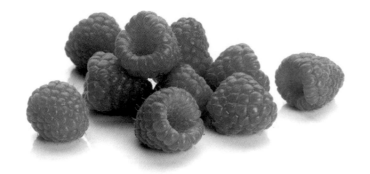

A Healthy Life—
body, mind, and spirit—
IS PART OF GOD'S PURPOSE FOR YOU!

Siloam brings you books, e-books, and other media from trusted authors on today's most important health topics. Check out the following links for more books from specialists such as *New York Times* best-selling author Dr. Don Colbert and get on the road to great health.

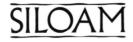

Ignite Your SPIRITUAL HEALTH
with these FREE Newsletters

CHARISMA HEALTH
Get information and news on health-related topics and studies, and tips for healthy living.

POWER UP! FOR WOMEN
Receive encouraging teachings that will empower you for a Spirit-filled life.

CHARISMA MAGAZINE NEWSLETTER
Get top-trending articles, Christian teachings, entertainment reviews, videos and more.

CHARISMA NEWS WEEKLY
Get the latest breaking news from an evangelical perspective every Monday.

SIGN UP AT:
nl.charismamag.com

CHARISMA MEDIA